Medical Technology in JAPAN

Medical Technology in JAPAN

The Politics of Regulation

Christa Altenstetter

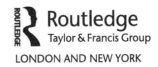

Routledge
Taylor & Francis Group

LONDON AND NEW YORK

Library of Congress Catalog Number: 2014005889

Library of Congress Cataloging-in-Publication Data

Altenstetter, Christa, author.
  Medical technology in Japan / by Christa Altenstetter.
    p. ; cm.
  Includes bibliographical references.
  ISBN 978-1-4128-5461-0 (alk. paper)
  I. Title.
  [DNLM: 1. Biomedical Technology--legislation & jurisprudence--Japan. 2. Biomedical Research--Japan. 3. Diffusion of Innovation--Japan. 4. Equipment and Supplies--standards--Japan. 5. Government Regulation--Japan. 6. Health Policy--Japan. W 32.5 JJ3]
  R853.C55
  610.72'40952--dc23
                                                            2014005889
ISBN 13: 978-1-4128-5461-0 (hbk)

Contents

List of Tables

Acknowledgments

I wish to acknowledge the financial support by the Japan Foundation Center for Global Partnership and the Social Science Research Council for an Abe Fellowship during my sabbatical in 2006–2007. I want to thank the Tokyo branch of the Japan Foundation Center for Global Partnership, especially Frank Baldwin and Takuya Toda for facilitating the field research, and Eric A. Feldman, Robert B. Leflar, and Marc A. Rodwin, all members of the United Kingdom-Japan-United States network (UJU), for their help in getting me started by putting me in touch with academics in the USA and Japan. Support for this project was also provided by a PSC-CUNY Award, jointly funded by the Professional Staff Congress and the City University of New York, 2011–2013.

Thanks to the support of Professor Takeshi Igarashi from the Graduate School of Law and Politics at the University of Tokyo, I had office space, Internet access, library privileges, and, most importantly, access to the University of Tokyo Hospital outpatient facility as well as the Student Health Center during my two stays in Tokyo. I benefited greatly from Professor Norio Higushi's large network of legal scholars and contacts in Tokyo and Japan, and from the wise counsel of Professors Naoki Ikegami (Department of Health Policy and Management at Keio University), Kazuhiro Sase (Clinical Pharmacology, Yutendo University School of Medicine), Yoshihiro Arakawa (The University of Tokyo Hospital), Toshihiko Hasegawa (Nippon Medical School), Koichi Kawabuchi (Tokyo Medical and Dental University), Teruo Okano (Institute of Advanced Biomedical Engineering and Science, Tokyo Women's Medical University), Tomonori Hasegawa (Toho University School of Medicine), Akira Akabayashi (Graduate School of Medicine, The University of Tokyo), Kazutomo Minami (Nihon University), and Takahiro Ueyama (Sophia University).

Although it may be due to the newness of the research on medical devices in Japan, in the three months that I spent as a visiting professor at the University of Tokyo's Graduate School of Law and Politics, I did not meet a single Japanese interlocutor or a social science scholar who had a remote interest in or knowledge about the politics and policy processes clustering around medical technologies. A good many Japanese contacts in other universities, institutions, and companies helped early on to guide me to the proper contacts and organizations. I had early contacts with Professors Naoki Ikegami and John Creighton Campbell, two of Japan's leading scholars on health policy. Professor Naoki Ikegami managed to get a personal invitation for me to attend the international conference *Leadership Dialogue for Stakeholders and Policy Leaders from Japan and the United States*, in Karuizawa, Japan, on April 21–23, 2007. This was a unique opportunity for participant observation and collection of empirical data, including establishing contacts with the experts, for which I am grateful. I was also fortunate to establish contact with Professor Norio Higuchi, University of Tokyo Law School, through the UJU network; he graciously offered his extensive network of scholars, lawyers, and collaborators for further contacts. Professors Robert B. Leflar and Marc A. Rodwin, also members of the UJU network, provided precious advice. Without the UJU network, initiated and run by Adam Oliver of the London School of Economics and Political Science, this study would never have started. Thank you for the generosity of time, patience, and help in completing this study.

Many thanks also to Shiomi Kasahara, a former student of the Political Science Department at the Graduate School and University Center of the City University of New York, who translated Japanese-language internal memos, government documents, and other primary materials. I would also like to thank Shigehiro Suzuki for his translations of passages from Japanese books, and Patricia Stapleton for her diligent, responsible, and constructive assistance with the drafts of this manuscript.

Finally, I want to thank all who made themselves available for interviews, despite busy schedules, though the remaining interviewees must remain unnamed. However, all errors of interpretation and assessment are solely mine.

Abbreviations

510(k)	Premarket notification (USA)
AAA	Abdominal aorta aneurysma
ACCJ	American Chamber of Commerce in Japan (known as American Medical Devices and Diagnostics Manufacturers' Association since April 1, 2009)
AdvaMed	The Advanced Medical Technology Association
AER	Adverse event reporting
AMDDMA	American Medical Devices and Diagnostics Manufacturers' Association
AVM	Arteriovenous malformation
BMS	Bare metal stent
BSI	British Standardization Institution
CAB	Conformity assessment body
CBER	Center for Biologics Evaluation and Research (USA)
CDRH	Center for Devices and Radiological Health (USA)
CE-marking	Certifying conformity with the essential requirements
CEN	European Committee for Standardisation
CENELEC	European Committee for Electrotechnical Standardisation
CEO	Chief executive officer
CME	Continued medical education
CRF	Case Report Form
CRO	Clinical research organization
CT	Computerized tomography
CTIRC	Clinical Trial Issue Review Committee
DES	Drug-eluting stent
DPC	Diagnostic procedure combination
DPJ	Democratic Party of Japan

DRGs	Diagnostic-related groups
EBC	European Business Council
EC(s)	Ethical committee(s)
EEC	European Economic Committee
EN	European Norm
ETP	European Executive Training Program
EU	European Union
EUCOMED	European Trade Association of the Medical Technology Industry
FAP	Foreign Average Pricing, also called the Foreign Reference Price system
FDA	Food and Drug Administration
GCP	Good clinical practice
GDP	Gross Domestic Product
GHTF	Global Harmonization Task Force
GIP	Good import practice
GKV	Gesetzliche Krankenversicherung (Statutory public health insurance)
GLP	Good laboratory practice
GMDC	Global Medical Device Conference
GMDN	Global Medical Device Nomenclature
GMO	Genetically modified organism
GMP	Good manufacturing practice
GPSP	Good post-marketing study practice
GQP	Good quality practice
GVP	Good vigilance practice
HAMTS	Highly advanced medical technology system
HBD	Harmonization-by-doing
HIB	Health Insurance Bureau
HIMA	Health Industry and Manufacturing Association
HIV	Human Immunodeficiency Virus
HPB	Health Policy Bureau
HRPPPs	Human Research Participant Protection Programs
HTA	Health Technology Assessment
IABP	Intra-aortic balloon pump
IDC	International Disease Classification
ICH	International Conference on Harmonization of Technical Requirements for Registration of Pharmaceuticals for Human Use

IEC	International Electrotechnical Commission
IMCJ	Internal Medical Center in Japan
IMDRF	International Medical Device Regulatory Forum
IND	Investigational new drug
IRB	Institutional Review Board
ISO	International Standards Organization
ISO-TC	International Standards Organizations, Technical Group
ISO-TC 210	Quality Management of Medical Devices
ISTAHC	International Society of Technology Assessment in Health Care
IT	Information Technology
IVDs	In vitro diagnostic products
JAAME	Japan Association for the Advancement of Medical Equipment
JACR	Japan Association of Clinical Reagents Industries
JAMEI	The Japan Assocation of Medical Equipment Industries
JCQHC	Japan Council for Quality Health Care
JETRO	Japan External Trade Organization
JFMDA	Japan Federation of Medical Device Associations
JIRA	The Japan Association of Radiological Systems
JISC	Japanese Industrial Standard Committee
JMA	Japan Medical Association
JMACCT	Japan Medical Association Center for Clinical Trials
JPHA	Japan Public Health Association
JTEC	Japan Tissue Engineering Corporation (near Nagoya)
LDP	Liberal Democratic Party
LOS	Length of stay
LTC	Long-term care
MAH	Market authorization holder
MD&D	Medical Device & Diagnostic Subcommittee (ACCJ)
METI	Ministry of Economics, Trade, and Industry
MEXT	Ministry of Education, Culture, Sports, Science, and Technology
MHLW	Ministry of Health, Labor, and Welfare
MTLF	Medical Technology Leadership Forum
MHW	Ministry of Health and Welfare
MITI	Ministry of International Trade and Industry
MOFA	Ministry of Foreign Affairs

MOSS	Market-oriented, sector-selective talks
MOU	Memorandum of understanding
MRA	Mutual recognition agreement
MRI	Magnetic resonance imaging
NCAR	National Competent Authority Report
NDA	New Drug Application
NPU	National Policy Unit, Cabinet Secretariat
NTB	Non-tariff barriers
OECD	Organization for Economic Cooperation and Development
OPSR	Organization for Pharmaceutical Safety and Research
PAB	Pharmaceutical Affairs Bureau
PAL	Pharmaceutical Affairs Law
PARI	Policy Alternatives Research Institute
PBM	Pacific Bridge Medical
PET	Positron emission tomography
PFSB	Pharmaceutical Food and Safety Bureau
PMA	Premarket approval
PMDA	Pharmaceuticals and Medical Device Agency
PMDEC	Pharmaceutical and Medical Devices Evaluation Center
PMDL	Pharmaceutical and Medical Devices Law (prior to 2013 PAL)
PMS	Postmarket surveillance
PTCA	Percutaneous transluminal coronary angioplasty
QAL	Quality of life
QMS	Quality management system
RAJ	Regulatory Affairs Journal
R&D	Research and development
RAPS	Regulatory Affairs Professional Society
R-zone	Reasonable allowance (margin)
SEA	Single European Act
SG	Study group
SHI	Social health insurance
SOPs	Standard operating procedures
STED	Summary Technical Document for Demonstrating Conformity to the Essential Principles of Safety and Performance of Medical Devices (abbreviated as STED) for Japan, the European Union, the United States of America, and Australia

STMs	Special treatment materials, or special treatment medical devices (Nakatoni)
TÜV	Technischer Überwachungsverein
UJU	United Kingdom-Japan-United States electronic network
UK MHRA	United Kingdom Medicines and Healthcare Products Regulatory Agency
USITC	US International Trade Commission
USTR	US trade representative
US (510(k))	Refers to the article in the 1976 Medical Devices Amendments
WG	Working group
WHO	World Health Organization
WTO	World Trade Organization

Japanese terms

Amakudari	"Descended from heaven," literally translated, also known as revolving door politics
Chuikyo	The Central Social Insurance Medical Council
Debaisū-ragū	Device lag
Gaiyo	STED
Hiyari hatto	Adverse event reporting
Iyaku-bugaihin	Quasi-drugs or generics
Kento kaigai	Study groups
Kenporen	The representation of self-insured private sector employers
Keidanren	Japan Federation of Economic Organizations
Nikkeiren	Japan Federation of Employers Association Keidanren and Nikkeiren merged in May 2002
Shingikai	The politics of consultation and advice giving by advisory councils and committees
Shonin	Product approval dossier
Tachiai	Mutual dependence in supplier-purchaser relationship
Zoku	Tribe

1

Introduction

Japan suffers from a severe medical device lag, including *in vitro* diagnostic products (IVDs). This lag is conventionally understood as the absence of treatment and procedures that are available to patients in Europe and the United States on average three to five years earlier than in Japan. The lag can alternatively be described as treatment obtained only after considerable delays. To remedy this deficit, the Japanese government has engaged in building regulatory capacity, reorganizing existing regulatory structures, and bettering its medical-clinical infrastructures through a variety of initiatives, programs, and actions since 2005. Reform is ongoing.

This study seeks to explain the driving forces that have shaped medical technology regulations (both on paper and in practice), how and why these forces differ from other nations, and how and why they have changed in recent years. To do so, it integrates a theoretical approach with historical assumptions about how institutions evolve: how they change, resist change, or adjust and transform to meet new circumstances and developments (Thelen, 2003: 208–240; Hall, 2003: 373–404; Pierson and Skocpol, 2002: 693–721). Thelen also speaks to "mechanisms of institutional reproduction" (2003: 210–211) and "institutional layering." The research found several traces of institutional reproduction and layering on several administrative levels: both at the macro and micro levels of the Japanese political-administrative system. Depending on the regulatory issue under consideration, some tools have substantial implications for the practice of medicine, the delivery of health services, and the use of medical devices in diagnosis and treatment, including clinical research. Several distinct but interlinked narratives will be offered explaining why Japanese patients have not benefited from the revolutionary advances of medical technologies of the last two decades, and why they are still disadvantaged compared to their American and European cousins. To provide the political and institutional context of medical technology regulation, the study draws on an extensive reading of scholarship in three disciplines (government and politics—including health policy analysis—law, and medicine). These sources provide valuable institutional and organizational foundations for this study of regulatory policy on medical devices in Japan.

Power and lobbying merit close attention. Yet reducing explanations to politics alone is simplistic. Knowing the content of regulatory policy and taking into account an array of highly complicated substantive details are necessary before any meaningful assessments of Japanese regulatory practices can be offered. Most relevant substantive details for achieving the twin objectives of medical technology regulation—reviewing and approving medical devices for trade while also securing patient safety concerns and releasing them for treatment in a timely fashion—are buried under layers upon layers of rules, technical details, and legal codes.

From the theoretical perspective of historical institutionalism, medical device regulatory policy is embedded in culture, law, and institutions both at the macro and the micro levels of the political system. This perspective also has implications for the advisory council and scientific committees and how they are anticipated to provide domain knowledge and expertise and hence contribute to the final decisions on regulatory policy of medical technologies. To set the stage for the recent regulatory developments and activities in the device sector in Japan in recent years, I show how the medical device-specific regulatory institutions have evolved in Japan; how they have changed since 2005 when PAL, the most important legislative project for drugs and medical devices, was adopted; and how and why these institutions and routines are different from those in the United States and the European Union.

The literature on comparative health-care reform (Marmor et al., 2005, 2009; Marmor and Wendt, 2011; Tuohy, 1999; "Legacies and latitude in European health policy," 2005) and drug regulation is substantial, yet little research has provided comparative analyses of medical devices. The argument is often made that medical device regulation "is too technical" (Interview #8) and, by implication, of little interest to the social science community. This commentary is not convincing. How do we know what the conflicts among various parties are all about and why they arise, unless we disentangle the layers of technical norms and legal procedures and identify the various professional, political, and bureaucratic "mechanisms of institutional reproduction" (Thelen, 2003: 210–211) and channels of communication? On the other hand, law has largely disappeared from the mainstream curriculum of political science and public policy, despite Theodore J. Lowi's (1972; 1973) early invitation to public policy scholars to not only ask what is policy as policy (government intentions), but also what is policy as law (procedures). Given the technological complexity of the subject matter and the high product differentiation, ignoring "technical details" is not an option.[1] Neither can the various political and institutional factors that impact regulatory policymaking in Japan be ignored.

Most laypeople, regardless of whether they live in the United States, Japan, or Europe, are unaware of the range of medical devices, their multiple uses, and their benefits to patients and physicians in diagnosis and treatment, including the implantation of devices into the human body. This is why the first task requires identifying the descriptive characteristics of medical devices, the regulatory framework of medical devices, and the industrial sub-sector of medical devices, as well as clarifying technical issues. Drugs and medical devices share one property: they interact with the human body; but all common properties end there.

A hospital management expert and long-time observer of health-care delivery in Japan (Interview #43) explained five distinct properties of medical devices that drugs do not have. These properties merit close attention because they clarify why medical devices are not drugs. First, a medical device can be implanted in the body and is not supposed to leave the body, such as an artificial knee, hip, or breast implant. Second, a medical device can be in the body but is ultimately removable based on the doctor's judgment, such as a screw. Third, a medical device can be in the body only temporarily (about five or ten minutes), such as a suture used during a procedure. Fourth, a medical device can touch the body and transmit energy, such as a thermal bandage. Finally, a medical device can either touch the body or collect information, such as a stethoscope.

From the above, it is obvious why physicians and surgeons play such an important role in patient outcomes apart from patients themselves, and why medical devices should not be treated as if they were drugs. Table 1.1 illustrates the broad spectrum of medical devices where individual devices make contributions distinct from drugs to health and patient outcomes and whose function and risk levels vary enormously. Yet despite these differences, all medical devices and approximately 370 *in vitro* diagnostic products (IVDs) on the Japanese market are regulated under the drug regime.[2] The submission of medical technology regulation under the drug regulatory framework in Japan has been the target of severe and enduring complaints by domestic and foreign device makers alike.

Table 1.1. Examples of medical devices.

- Anesthetic machines and monitors
- Apnea monitors
- Artificial eyes
- Blood transfusion and filtration devices
- Breast implants
- Cardiac monitors
- Cardiopulmonary bypass devices
- Clinical thermometers
- Condoms
- Contact lenses and prescribable spectacles
- CT scanners
- Defibrillators
- Dental equipment and dentures
- Dental material and restoratives
- Diagnostic kits and tests
- Dialyzers
- Electrosurgery devices
- Endoscopes
- Enteral and parenteral feeding systems
- Equipment for disabled people
- Examination gloves
- Fetal monitors
- Hearing aids and inserts
- Heart valves
- Hospital beds
- Hydrocephalus shunts
- Incontinence pads and controllers
- Intrauterine devices
- Intravascular catheters and cannulae
- Lithotripters
- Medical lasers
- Medical textiles, dressings, hosiery, and surgical supports
- Laboratory equipment
- Operating tables

- Orthopedic implants
- Ostomy and incontinence appliances
- Pacemakers
- Physiotherapy equipment
- Prescribing footwear
- Pressure sore relief devices
- Radiotherapy machines
- Resuscitators
- Special support seating
- Sphygmomanometers
- Stents
- Suction devices
- Surgical instruments and gloves
- Sutures, clips, and staples
- Syringes and needles
- Ultrasound imagers
- Urinary catheters, vaginal speculae, and drainage bags
- Ventilators
- Walking aids
- Wheelchairs

Source: Health Industry Task Force (2004). Adapted from Fabio Pammolli et al., *Medical Devices: Competitiveness and Impact on Public Health Expenditure.* Competiveness, Markets and Regulation (CERM), Rome. Study prepared for the Directorate Enterprise of the European Commission. July 2005: 11.

From the above, it is clear that medical devices are definitely not pills, nor are they derivatives of drugs. Neither are the two industries structurally identical cases (Altenstetter and Permanand, 2007). Four structural differences between the two sectors need to be differentiated, as they are the source of distinct political dynamics in each sector: first, the dominance of globally operating multinational drug companies in contrast to a majority of small- and medium-sized device-making companies, in addition to a few globally operating device makers. Second, patenting drugs and patenting medical devices are functionally not identical. Patenting medical devices in their entirety is not possible; only the basic principles of a medical device are patentable and can be used in different applications. Third, the long-term research and development process of drugs and devices greatly differ: drug testing primarily occurs in a controlled environment *ex ante* and limited observations *ex post*. While this is not the case for medical devices, with limited *ex ante* clinical trials, the only way to establish safety, performance, and efficacy are *ex post* clinical trials. Fourth, the medical device innovation process is incremental by nature. For example, pacemakers or orthopedic implants are improved in small steps from one generation to the next. A note to readers: While those two terms, efficacy and efficiency, may at first appear to be synonymous and interchangeable; in fact, they are distinct constructs. Efficacy refers to health outcomes achieved under ideal laboratory conditions, while effectiveness recognizes that outcomes are achieved under routine clinical conditions.

Multiple Regulatory Policy Spaces

Medical technology regulation occupies several distinct policy spaces (a term coined by Hancher and Moran, 1989: 271–299)—the manufacture, trade, and use of medical devices in clinical practice—and it straddles the boundaries of several disciplines. The regulation of manufacturing and trading medical devices moves within narrowly defined parameters, but the use of medical devices relies on a combination of interconnected regulated activities: manufacturing, delivering health care, and the practice of clinical medicine, including the regulation of the medical profession. The effects of interactions between these associated policy and institutional legacies merit close attention.

To differentiate analytically between the effects of interaction among four major driving forces would be ideal: (i) the global market integration in medical goods and services; (ii) the dramatic and revolutionary technological and material innovations of the last twenty years that have improved the diagnostic capabilities but much less the treatment capabilities by medical professionals in most advanced societies, though much less so in Japan; (iii) an aging Japanese society that no longer blindly trusts its doctors as in the past but now expects and demands more; and (iv) the ways in which health care is delivered within an established health-care system. In reality, the lines between these sub-sectors are blurred in light of the many moving parts amidst elements of inertia and turf protection. To grasp medical technology regulation in all intertwined facets and fluid boundaries requires connecting the dots among distinct activities in separate venues, as chapters 2 through 9 will address.

Case Study Design

How and why regulation and health policy in the context of medical technology regulation must be brought together in one analytical framework is dictated by reality, but even policymakers are limited in their vision. As late as May 23, 2007, the Sixtieth World Health Assembly of the World Health Organization voted on a definition of health technology that exclusively focused on activities in the health-care system and clinical trials. "The term health technologies refers to the application of organized knowledge and skills in the form of devices, medicines, vaccines, procedures and systems developed to solve a health problem and improve quality of lives" (Sixtieth World Health Assembly, 2007: 1). This perspective, endorsed at the highest level of global health policymakers, is blind to the organizational and institutional contexts that serve as basic structural foundations for the delivery and regulation of treatment and the diagnosis of diseases.

A definition of regulation must be sensitive to concerns about risks to patients, not simply to the regulation of products. A broader definition is as follows:

> Technology in health care can be defined as the stock of usable knowledge regarding healthcare treatment that is incorporated in drugs, devices and medical and surgical procedures used in medical care as in the organizational and supportive systems within which such care is delivered . . . Applied more narrowly to medical devices, this reference definition covers not only innovation in the *products/devices,* but also in the *processes* for their use (new surgical procedures), as well as in the *skills* and support systems through which they are operated and dispensed. (Pammolli, 2005: 38)[3]

Another concept requires definition. It is the concept "life cycle" or "life span," conventionally understood as covering rules and procedures in the pre-market and post-market phases. In reality, this concept has two distinct uses. First, it stands for an analytical framework that accounts for the stakeholders who discuss, debate, and evaluate topics on risk regulation and independent scientific advice and assessment ranging from broad to very specific technical issues. Second, the concept also stands for the assignment of responsibilities to stakeholders and policy actors in particular phases of the regulatory process, both *ex ante* and *ex post,* and for the protection of certain rights.

The written and oral sources used in this research help to unearth strong evidence that pressures for change originated from within and, above all, from outside Japan in three distinct areas: the delivery of health care, clinical medicine, and the regulatory framework (narrowly defined). Chief among the internal pressures are continually rising health-care costs, an aging population, and inadequacy of a regulatory pathway for medical devices under the drug framework, as well as the shadow of past scandals over HIV-infected blood products (Feldman, 1999: 59–93) and the ten thousand hepatitis C patients infected by tainted blood between 1970 and 1990 (*The Japan Times*, January 16, 2008; *Asahi Shimbun*, January 12–13, 2008). Medical errors and litigation are increasingly public knowledge, and the Japanese now have higher expectations about the health care they receive today than a decade ago. Finally, the restructuring of regulatory functions in the Ministry of Health, Labor, and Welfare (MHLW) and the Pharmaceutical and Medical Devices Agency (PMDA) in recent years is a direct response to external pressures for change and improvement of, first, the review and approval procedures and processes of medical devices and, second, lowering the persistent price controls and raising the reimbursement levels of medical technologies. Japan's dependence on the United States has also contributed to domestic pressures to make Japan more autarkic and not as dependent on the United States as in the past.

Japan depends heavily on US-manufactured medical devices. Over 50 percent of all devices used in Japan are imported from the United States, a number that has steadily risen from 35.5 percent in 1995 and 45 percent in 2003 (Hiroshi Yamamoto, 2005). According to one informant (Interview #57), Japan imports 80 percent of all catheters and 100 percent of pacemakers from the United States or Europe. The United States government, the European Union, and vested interests of the US-led med-tech industry have put enormous pressures on the Japanese government since the 1990s (USITC, 2007). The external and internal driving forces, taken together, add weight to the basic premises and key arguments I develop in this work.

Methods and Data Collection

This qualitative case study draws on interviews, field observations, and document analysis, including industry newsletters and websites, to get information and gain an understanding of how regulatory policy is formulated and implemented today. To establish the macro-political and historical-institutional context, it relies heavily on secondary scholarship in three disciplinary fields: government and politics, including health policy analysis, law, and medicine. The case study is designed to give voice to individuals and experts actively involved in domestic regulatory processes and to learn about their experience with regulatory policy, its application, and their participation in international processes on the harmonization of medical device regulations. They are well acquainted with the contextual conditions and the political and administrative rationales of regulation in Japan. Awareness of these conditions helps to understand and develop an appreciation for how Japanese officials, experts, and members of academia (including American and Japanese business interests) tend to view, assess, and experience the policies and activities of their own governments. Said differently, listening to their explanations of how they are affected by the Pharmaceutical Affairs Law (PAL) is a valuable source of information, in addition to lengthy quotes from published materials, which compensate for missing empirical data in Japan. Japan thus represents "the perfect case of 'experimental' variation" (Schwartz and Pharr, 2003: 6).

Over sixty semi-structured interviews were conducted with officials of MHLW and staff of PMDA, academics in various disciplines, senior and junior physicians, medical and engineering scientists, and American and Japanese representatives of device-making companies and sectoral trade associations. Informants were questioned about their experience with PAL after 2005. All interviews were transcribed and coded to protect the privacy of the informants, unless explicit permission to quote was given. The interview data were triangulated with scholarship in three related fields and information obtained from trade journals and e-newsletters of regulatory professional societies. Trade journals and e-newsletters are crucial for the "technical details" of regulation and, importantly, for updating the study to the beginning of 2014. Shiomi Kasahara, a former political science graduate student at the Graduate School and University Center of the City University of New York (CUNY), translated Japanese-language internal memos, government documents, and other primary materials such as memos and notes received during interviews in 2008. In 2010, Shigehiro Suzuki, a doctoral student from the same program, translated passages from Japanese books. Together, the interviews and research materials form the scholarly foundation of this monograph.

Medical Technology Regulation

The objective of medical technology regulation, consistent with regulatory science (Yeo, 2010: 1),[4] is to minimize risks to patients/consumers by securing high quality and efficient medical technologies, while also protecting property rights and creating a level playing field in an open market and promoting the competitiveness of the Japanese industry in international trade. Qualitatively and theoretically, these objectives require a delicate balancing act between patient and user safety, on the one hand, and the commercialization of medical innovations, trade, and profits on the other. For patient safety, a dual and complex balancing act exists between granting early access to new and promising medical devices and securing appropriate guarantees on safety and quality. With the rapid innovations of the last two decades, an increasingly globalizing marketplace, and aggressive trade and fierce competition, finding the right balance between early release and medical device safety, efficacy, and effectiveness has become more complex than thirty years ago.

The rapid and revolutionary advances in science, knowledge, and new applications in medicine, including in information technology (IT), materials, and genetics in medical practice during the last two decades, have placed Japan at the center of an array of paradoxes. Each paradox likely stems from a combination of different contributing factors, but taken together these tend to reinforce the negative effects of each. The first paradox is that while the Japanese have universal access to health care (unlike their American counterparts, but like their European cousins) and the longest life expectancy in the world, their access to advanced medical technologies is more limited than access to medical technologies in Europe and the United States (USITC, 2007). For example, "an advanced pacemaker for cardiac resynchronization therapy was available to patients in Europe in 2001 and the United States in 2003, and [was] only available to Japan in August 2006" (Ludwig, 2006). In an interview with Alex Wood in 2007, Derrick Buddles,[5] speaking for the ACCJ's Medical Devices and Diagnostic Subcommittee (MD&D)[6] in Tokyo, explained the latest developments in Japan:

> The development is largely the product of a growing realization by the media and the public that new technologies and product improvements take much longer to reach Japanese patients than those overseas . . . According to a ACCJ study, "Japanese patients have access only to about half of the products or brands available to those in the US or Europe . . . As this awareness has grown it has

turned a spotlight on the role of elected politicians in ensuring that new technologies are made available both as safely as possible and as quickly as possible." (Buddles as quoted in Wood, 2007)

A second paradox concerns the distance between the progress in cell and tissue engineering[7] and other fields of medicine,[8] with Japanese scientists among those recognized for prestigious awards like Nobel prizes, and the low development, production, and commercialization of medical devices and limited diffusion of advanced treatment products (Foreign Press Center Japan, 2007: 103–108). The third paradox is that Japan not only lags behind other advanced industrialized societies in terms of patient access to the latest innovations on average by three to five years, but Japan also lags behind even other Asian countries, such as China, India, and Thailand (Gross and Hirose, 2009). Lengthy approval processes mean higher costs for the US-led medical technology industry, which must keep out-of-date product lines just for Japan (AdvaMed, October 24, 2007). These "Japan-only-products" are mostly orthopedic devices and heart valves but not exclusively (Interview #52). A fourth paradox is the existence in Japan of high-quality and state-of-the-art technology that made the Japanese electronics and car industries famous. Yet this position is not replicated in biotechnology, clinical research, or health care. There is no "Toyota" of medicine and health services in Japan. Finally, economic and fiscal constraints resulting from a stagnant economy since the 1990s forced the Japanese government to pursue a policy of cost containment in health care while neglecting a strategy of facilitating access to medical technologies and investing and modernizing an underdeveloped medical technology sector.

Health policy scholars have reacted to rising costs in the health-care sector by searching for solutions based on a mix of retaining an egalitarian ethos but increasing co-payments or introducing market principles in health-care reform (discussed in Chapter 2). While Japanese health policy analysts disagree on whether access to new medical devices and advanced medical treatments is subordinate to cost-containment policies, from the perspective of this study this interpretation is plausible and on target. Indeed, Japanese health policy analysts are committed to universal health insurance, but they approach health-care reform through their preferred lenses of how the system should and could be organized and reorganized, financed, and improved: that is, a commitment to public health insurance with a minimum of market principles integrated into it, or a commitment to reforms that are augmented with market-oriented elements.

Finally, Japan suffers from a shortage of staff knowledgeable in advanced therapies and medical innovations. This presents the Ministry of Health, Welfare, and Labor (MHLW) and the regulatory authority, the Pharmaceutical and Medical Devices Agency (PMDA), with major challenges. How can decision-makers act and regulate on the basis of the latest know-how of medical-technological innovations when they do not have basic knowledge and skills themselves? Who has domain knowledge and experience, and where does scientific advice come from? Chapters 4 through 6 will discuss these issues.

Demographics

Compared to Western societies, Japan has the highest percentage of its population at sixty-five years and older. In theory, they would benefit from all kinds of coronary stenting and advanced new treatments for cardiovascular diseases, as well as from new orthopedic advancements and ortho technologies. In a comparative perspective, taking population size into consideration, the differences are even more apparent: Japan had about 128 million inhabitants over the age of sixty-five (over 22 percent of its population) in 2007, while Germany, with 82 million inhabitants, had less than 20 percent over the age of sixty-five in 2009, the highest in Europe. The percentages have not changed since 2007 (OECD, 2011a; 2011b). Moreover, the Japanese population is reported as aging more rapidly than a few Western societies, such as the UK, France, Germany, Sweden, and the United States (OECD, 2010; Wilkinson, 2007: 98). It has the highest projected share of the population at eighty-plus years (OECD, 2011b).

According to conventional wisdom, healthy, active, and independent aging usually generates demands for medical technologies (WHO Western Pacific Region, 2010). Japan is richly endowed with medical technologies in the area of imaging devices (MRI and CT) and renal dialysis, which stem from domestic production. Interestingly, the level of technology penetration by far exceeds that of European countries and the United States (Pammolli et al., 2005: 24). More exactly, according to a Japanese source, 23 percent of hospitals have a capability for magnetic resonance imaging, 27 percent for angiography, and 72 percent for fiberscopes for the upper gastrointestinal tract (Tatara and Okamoto, 2009: 87). Tellingly, this record is not matched in all fields of clinical medicine due to inadequate resources, skilled capabilities, and limited access to new therapies with advanced devices. This record largely explains why the Japanese have become dissatisfied with their health-care system lately (discussed in Chapter 2).

In light of the highest life expectancy in Japan among all industrialized societies, the argument could be made that Japan does not really need advanced technologies. Yet this line of reasoning is not tenable. It is not known how many Japanese who live a long life are handicapped, in wheelchairs, or suffering from treatable conditions and chronic disease and could be helped by innovative medical treatments with new devices. However, Japan has the longest stay in hospitals among all advanced societies. John Campbell and Naoki Ikegami (2009) present data that show that Japanese patients are hospitalized instead of receiving long-term care at home or living in nursing homes. Rodwin and Gusmano's work (2006) on the elderly in Japan also lends support to dismiss the argument that because the Japanese have the longest longevity, there is no need and demand for new innovative medical treatments (Gusmano et al., 2010).

For causes of mortality, Japan has a record similar to other advanced societies, with cancer ranking first, followed by heart and cerebrovascular disease (Kondo, 2007a; Kondo, 2006). The frequency of heart disease has increased by 23 percent and cancer by 22 percent from 1995 to 2005 (Kondo 2006). This rise in cardiovascular disease is one of the reasons why some progress to close the medical device "lag" has been possible in the last few years through a variety of strategic measures: (i) the acceleration of the approval route for the most-needed treatments; (ii) cooperation in global joint and cardiovascular clinical trials and participating in harmonization-by-doing (HBD) pilot projects (Chapter 7); and (iii) modest investment in the health technology sector (Chapter 6).

Cardiology: A Test Case

On January 25, 2008, I interviewed Dr. Kazutomo Minami in Tokyo, where he served as the head of the Department of Cardiovascular Surgery at Nihon University School of Medicine. He has acquired over thirty years of experience as a cardiologist-surgeon in Germany, and has authored a comparative study on cardiology in Japan and Germany (2004). According to Dr. Minami, Japanese cardiologists use third-generation pacemakers, whereas their peers in Europe and the United States may receive the latest, and in most cases an improved, fifth- or sixth-generation implant. The latest technology is not always the best and most efficacious. But a pacemaker that uses bulky technology and is highly inconvenient to the patient is less desirable for implantation than a significantly slimmer and incrementally improved version. In vascular surgery, the delays in market approval are said to be even longer. For example, stent grafts for abdominal aorta aneurysma

(AAA) were approved in the EU in 1997, and then two years later in the United States, but not until 2006 in Japan (Ohki, 2007).

Dr. Minami also explained a fundamental difference in medical culture and training in Japan compared to surgical practice in the West. Surgeons in medical schools in Japan used to be promoted exclusively on the basis of scientific publications rather than surgical skills and experience. Hardly anyone would question the proposition that experience and surgical skills are the best resource a surgeon can have. Thirty years ago, Dr. Minami's mentor told him, "No matter how many patients you see overseas, and no matter how good you are with your surgical techniques, unless you publish a paper, you won't get a job when you get back to Japan" (2004: 64). Dr. Minami stayed abroad and made his professional career as a cardiovascular surgeon in Germany. Little has changed since he started his career thirty years ago, except for a few modest changes such as the mandatory internships and specialty training introduced in 2004 (discussed in Chapter 6).

In his book (2004), Dr. Minami compared the number of heart surgeries performed in Germany, where he spent his career as a cardiologist, and in the United States to the biggest facility in Japan. Over six thousand cases per year were performed at the Center of Heart Disease in Germany (Düsseldorf, later Bad Neuhausen) and four thousand cases were performed at a large facility in the United States, compared to eight hundred cases at the biggest facility in Japan (2004: 25–26). Heart surgeries in Japan are done in all kinds of very small and large hospitals, with a frequency of surgery ranging from a high number per year to a very few surgeries in a small hospital per year (tables 1.2 and 1.3).

Table 1.2. Facilities where heart operations are performed: Japan and Germany.

Japan (533 facilities)	Germany (82 facilities)
Less than 100 heart operations— 118 facilities (24 %)	Less than 1000 heart operations— 2 (13%)
100–199 operations—198 facilities (41%)	1000–1999 operations—43 (47%)
200–299 operation—198 facilities (25%)	2000–2999 operations—32 (35 %)
300–399 operations—33 facilities (7%)	3000–3999 operations—4 (4%)
More than 400 operations— 17 facilities (3%)(1%)	More than 4000 operations—1

Source: Kazutomo Minami, *Konna Iryoude Iidesuka: Nihonde Okonawareteiru Iryou, Doitsude Okonawareteiru Iryou* (translated as *Is This Medical Care Good Enough? Medical Care in Japan and Germany.* Haru Shobo, Tokyo, 2004, table (chart 2), p. 53.

Table 1.3. Number of heart operations performed by trainees (less than 6 years of experience) and surgeons (from 7 to 10 years of experience) in Japan.

I. Overall	II. Less than 6 years of experience	III. More than 7 years of experience
- 0 Operations: 130 (25%)	- 0 Operations: 116 (46%)	- 0 Operations: 15 (5%)
- 1–5 Operations: 107 (21%)	- 1–5 Operations: 66 (27%)	- 1–5 Operations: 41 (15%)
- 6–10 Operations: 52 (10%)	- 6–10 Operations: 27 (11%)	- 6–10 Operations: 25 (9%)
- 11–20 Operations: 84 (16%)	- 11–20 Operations: 23 (9%)	- 11–20 Operations: 61 (23%)
- 21–50 Operations: 87 (17%)	- 21–50 Operations: 10 (4%)	- 21–50 Operations: 77 (28%)
- More than 51 Operations: 59 (11%)	- More than 51 Operations: 7 (3%)	- More than 51 Operations: 52 (19%)

Sources: The Japanese Association for Thoracic Surgery, November 2003, p.81. *Source:* Kazutomo Minami, *Konna Iryoude Iidesuka: Nihonde Okonawareteiru Iryou, Doitsude Okonawareteiru Iryou* (translated as *Is This Medical Care Good Enough? Medical Care in Japan and Germany.* Haru Shobo, Tokyo, 2004, table (chart 5), p. 81.

The Attractiveness of the Japanese Market

The Japanese market is the third largest market for medical devices and the second largest market for most US companies. According to JETRO, the Japan external trade organization, US companies receive approval for their devices in Japan on average 2.5 years after receiving approval in the United States. Delays are costly. Medical devices have a short life span (of between eighteen to thirty-six months maximum). Device makers, on average, attempt to recover costs on the market during this period, unlike in the drug sector where the cost of R&D can be recuperated over the life of the drug's patent life. Why Japan's proactive state, which has taken the lead in other sectors of the economy, has not engaged in providing leadership and vision in modernizing medicine, medical education, and clinical research remains a fundamental puzzle. Chapters 5 and 6 attempt to answer this puzzle. Japan suffers from an inability to create innovative products in a weak medical technology sector. Japan's failure to invest R&D in the medical technology sector in the past has created a considerable disadvantage today.

How does the Japanese market compare to the markets in the European Union and the United States? Table 1.4 clearly shows the dominance of the US industry on the international market in terms of product sectors, size, and employment, in comparison to the European Union and Japan.

Table 1.4. The Japanese medical device sector in comparative perspective.

Medical devices	United States	EU	Japan
Production ■ Global share ■ Value (2005) ■ Dominant products	51% $92.0 billion - Interventional cardiology (coronary stents, Pacemakers, defibrillators) - Diagnostic imaging - Orthopedic implants - Patient monitoring - Medical and surgical instruments - In vitro diagnostics (IVD)	30% $38.0 billion - Diagnostic imaging - IVD - Orthopedic implants - Dialysis - Commodity hospital supplies	10% $14.2 billion (2004) - Diagnostic imaging - Optical (endoscopic) - Commodity hospital supplies
Consumption ■ Global share ■ Value (2005) ■ Population	50% $90.2 billion 298.4 million	30% $38.1 billion 457.0 million	10% $19.0 billion (2004) 127.5 million
Trade balance (2005)	$1.8 billion	$4.5 billion	$4.9 billion (2004)
Total Employment (2005)	388,400	393,000	68,000
National Health-care Expenditures (percent in GDP)	15%	7–8%	8%
Research & Development Expenditures*	10–13%	6%	6%

Source: United States International Trade Commission. *Medical Devices and Equipment: Competitive Conditions Affecting US Trade in Japan and Other Principal Foreign Markets.* Washington, DC: USITC, 2007: 3-2.
*Reported R&D expenditures as a share of sales.

Why does Japan lag behind other industrialized societies? Research indicates three preliminary explanations. The first explanation turns our attention to the chronic weakness of Japanese universities and medical schools, as both research institutions and as a recruitment place for young medical doctors to learn the skills of medical-clinical science in all its modern variations and specializations. Japanese medicine seems to remain embedded in the traditional paradigm of medicine and laboratory medical science of earlier periods and has not yet ventured into medicine of the twenty-first century.

A cross-national study of industrial sectors found that Japan also lagged behind in industries "involving chemistry, biotechnology, and other fields heavily dependent on basic science" compared to other social systems of production (Hollingsworth, 1997: 265–310). Knowledge and experience in these fields are vital ingredients for medical device innovations. Moreover, the number of new products developed by small firms was lowest in Japan as compared to four other advanced societies (Hollingsworth, 1997: 284). This low engagement is a serious drawback compared to very innovative small- and medium-sized companies in the United States and Europe. Hollingsworth's data are confirmed by a three-volume *History of Science and Technology in Contemporary Japan* (Nakayama et al., 2005a, 2005b, and 2006; and Bartholomew, 1989).

The medical profession and medical specialties are usually described as dynamic and entrepreneurial professions (Cohen and Hanf, 2004). These properties, individual exceptions notwithstanding, are practically absent in Japan. Lack of professional entrepreneurship and scientific curiosity has far-reaching implications for medicine, medical-technological innovations, and clinical research. This also has consequences for the review and registration of approved medical devices and their distribution and penetration into the health-care system, as well as their use.

Most laypersons perceive medicine as a universal science, but the practice of medicine largely depends on training, education, and the local culture of clinical practice (John E. Wennberg, the initiator of the Dartmouth Atlas of Health Care, 2008). This observation could not be more relevant than in the case of Japan. Medicine in Japan is local and inward looking. Specialty medicine in Japan has not evolved as in most other advanced societies. To the extent that it is practiced, it lacks standardized guidelines of good or best medical practice in most specialties, as discussed in Chapter 2.

A final but preliminary explanation of Japan's underdeveloped medical technology sector is that Japan historically has invested modest funding for medical research and R&D in medical technology. By contrast, the US medical technology industry is leading in this sector, having enjoyed a head start as a result of abundant venture capital, a social system of production that offers ample opportunities for small- and medium-sized device companies, and public funding of medical technology research in universities by the National Institutes of Health and other federal funding agencies (USITC, 2007: 2–5). By the same token, the European Union has made innovation and technology a priority of industrial policy, though with some delay compared to the United States. The EU promotes innovation by small- and medium-sized companies through a variety of initiatives.

From intensive study of English-language literature in three fields and three months of over sixty interviews with a cross-section of actors and actor groups, members of academia, and the health bureaucracy in Tokyo, a pattern of representative and self-reinforcing messages emerged that clearly justifies challenging the conventional wisdom that I heard repeatedly during the field research. Rather than solely blaming the bureaucracy, hidden protectionism, and an entrenched administrative culture for the delay of access to innovative technologies for Japanese patients (to repeat, five or six years in Japan compared to two in Europe and four in the United States), the evidence seems to point to three root causes for the current state of clinical research. First, the medical profession refuses to transition to a modern profession, to define itself in terms of professional autonomy in return for specified rights and obligations, and to provide guidance on the practice of medicine and specialty medicine following standardized procedures and standards of best practice (Freidson, 1970a and 1970b). A second structural feature is the relative weakness of both the Japanese medical technology sector and the biotechnology sector when compared to the pharmaceutical sector. A third factor is a lack of governmental vision and direction in advancing medicine in Japan and a reluctance, if not complicity, not to take on the all-powerful Japan Medical Association (JMA). No doubt, these various factors combine to account for the "device lag" and the unavailability of medical technologies in Japan as compared to other advanced societies. Deeply entrenched factors in industry, society, government, and medicine do not make for a favorable climate in the medical technology sector in Japan.

Within a six-month period, prior to and during my first stay in Tokyo in 2007, three events took place that provided rich empirical data reflecting the concerns of the US and Japanese policymaking and law-making communities. The first event, the so-called *Japan Submissions Workshop*, took place on November 8 and 9, 2006, in Tokyo and was organized by the US-based Advanced Medical Technology Association (AdvaMed). AdvaMed represents about five hundred med-tech companies operating in Japan and internationally. The conference materials form a good part of empirical information, in addition to information obtained through interviews. The second event was the *Japan-US HBD West 2007 Think Tank Meeting* on January 10 and 11, 2007, in Durham, North Carolina, followed by the *HBD East 2008 Think Tank Meeting* in Tokyo.[9] On April 21–23, 2007, these activities were topped by an international conference entitled *A Leadership Dialogue for Stakeholders and Policy Leaders from Japan and the United States*, sponsored by the US-based Medical Technology Leadership Forum (MTLF) based at the University of Minnesota. This conference was supported in name but not in funding by the US Department of Health and Human Services and the Ministry of Health, Labor, and Welfare of Japan in Karuizawa, Japan. This conference brought together all the relevant communities that have serious stakes in medical-technological innovations, their use in clinical practice, and regulations. Participants included American and Japanese government officials, elected politicians, officials from the Ministry of Health, Labor and Welfare (MHLW),[10] its Pharmaceutical and Food Safety Division (within MHLW), and the quasi-independent Pharmaceutical and Medical Devices Agency (PMDA). Among the invited guests were cardiovascular and orthopedic specialists and medical and biomedical scientists from the USA and Japan, including representatives of American trade groups as well as of individual American and Japanese companies.

A study of the Japanese system of medical device regulation is justified on several grounds. First, in 1992 Japan was among the founding members and early supporters of global harmonization[11] in the medical device sector along with the European Union (Altenstetter, 2008: 237–241), the United States, Australia, and Canada. The Global Harmonization Task Force (GHTF) brought together regulatory authorities and industry during the period of 1993 through early 2011, when it was replaced by the International Medical Device Regulatory Forum (IMDRF) as a regulators' forum only. Japan continues to be an active participant in the IMDRF.[12] Second, Japan is a favorite candidate for inclusion in cross-national social science research on advanced societies, despite the "uniquely unique" features of Japanese society and government (Lipset, 1996: 212). Is this characterization also valid for medical device regulation in Japan? Through historical and comparative references, I attempt to present comparative observations without intending to engage in a systematic cross-national comparison.

For historical-institutional context, I rely on scholarship in three disciplines that provide insights into the most striking contextual conditions. And I share Frank J. Schwartz's belief in the centrality of institutions. He writes,

> The most fundamental domestic determinants of economic policy are neither the rationality of monadic individuals [referring to the discussion of the decline of "Japan, Inc."], group dynamics, class struggles, nor national culture, but the institutions that mediate and structure the workings of those factors. The interests and ideas that drive policymaking are shaped, articulated, and advantaged—or disadvantaged—by the organization of a nation's state apparatus, electoral system, and private producer groups, for example. Of course, institutions constrain rather than single-handedly and deterministically cause political strategies and outcomes, and the same institutions that structure relations of power are themselves created and changed in political struggles. (Schwartz, 1998: xi)

This quote provides a valuable foundation to this investigation and the institutional configurations shaping, transforming, or resisting change. His portrayal of the workings of *shingikai*—also understood as the politics of consultation and advice giving—offers useful hints into how to interpret the lobbying of business interests and the influence of academic experts in committees or subcommittees advising the Cabinet, several offices in charge of medical technology regulation in MHLW or in PMDA, or *Chuikyo*, the most important advisory council and decision-making body for Japan's health insurance program, including the reimbursement of medical devices and price setting.

Preliminary findings suggest that medical device regulatory policy is framed, debated, and resolved under conditions of serious asymmetrical power relations among the health bureaucracy, business interests, and a scientifically disinclined lobby of the Japan Medical Association (JMA). Patient voices and participation of the public in medical technology regulation were largely absent, or at least until recently. Following the interpretation by health policy analysts and government specialists in Japan, an entrepreneurial medical profession in private practice has dominated the delivery of health care and has been complicit with the health bureaucracy in the Ministry of Health, Labor and Welfare (MHLW), while a clinically innovative but small medical scientific community has been sitting on the sidelines. This scenario has dominated medicine, medical research, and health care in Japan for several decades. Change is slow in coming.

For years the Ministry of Health, Labor, and Welfare, along with the Ministry of Finance and ultimately the Japanese government, have been interested in stemming the ever-rising tide of health-care costs. Reimbursement decisions of medical devices were subordinated to the logic of cost containment within the overall national budget over the last twenty years—an interpretation that is contested among Japanese health policy analysts. However, the evidence is strong to support alternative interpretations, as presented in Chapters 4 and 5.

Limitations of the Study

This study suffers from some limitations. A first limitation is one of language, which is shared with much social science writing in English. I began work on Japan without prior knowledge of the Japanese language, history, politics, or society. Instead, I draw on substantial English-language scholarship and primary government sources. The limitations are not fatal to the larger objectives of this study. They are offset by an abundance of interviews with informants from different realms of political life and the world of medical technologies in Tokyo. These local sources willingly shared their experiences and offered real-life and salient insights into the topic: social scientists, public health experts, and medical and pharmaceutical scientists, as well as government officials (MHLW and PMDA), lawyers, and representatives of American and Japanese businesses, including American and Japanese trade associations. Representing Japan in international meetings, workshops, and conferences, representatives of large Japanese device makers often translate Japanese legal texts and legislative drafts to the GHTF. A good number of medical-scientific and pharmaceutical experts I interviewed had studied and trained in the United States, including industry experts at business and management levels. A few had practiced in a medical specialty abroad, completing an entire professional career before returning to Japan, and had become much sought-after advisers to the government and the bureaucracy. English-language documentation can be found on the websites of the MHLW and the PMDA, although it is usually available only after a considerable delay of up to three years. Couched in flowery language, this documentation often does not specify the information that is relevant to drugs or to medical devices. In contrast, English-language e-newsletters by Pacific Bridge Medical (PBM), AdvaMed, the Regulatory Affairs Professional Society (RAPS), Eucomed's *What's New*, *Medical Product Outsourcing Magazine*, the Regulatory Affairs journal *Devices* (RAJDevices), and *Regulatory Affairs Medtech* (published by Informa, UK) inform about ongoing developments and provide valuable empirical data that are otherwise missing.

In this context, critical observers may raise questions whether the study gets the whole story. In defense, I conducted as many interviews with officials and advisers to the Cabinet or MHLW and academics as I did with industry insiders. In addition, academic scholarship in three disciplines guarded against one-sidedness and bias. This monograph is a first account of an empirical no-man's-land in Japan and could be of interest to a future research agenda for systematic study by Japanese social scientists.

Even the approximately sixty interviews conducted in Tokyo during my two stays totaling three months (April and May 2007 and January 2008) were exclusively conducted with English-speaking Japanese policymakers, experts, and contacts. A highly specialized terminology unique to this sector serves as *lingua franca* that is spoken and written in English. Most informants conversed in the *lingua franca*, which is preferable over grammatically correct translations but substantively incoherent texts.

At the end of my stay in Tokyo, I came away with the impression that most Japanese experts and individuals alike feel that Americans do not understand where the Japanese health-care system is coming from, what sustains it, or the historical commitment of the government to universal health care irrespective of means. In conversations with American contacts, what stood out and was critically commented on are the tremendous barriers to the Japanese market and the delayed use of high-tech medical devices in Japan, rather than Japan's achievement of having universal health care coverage. From an American perspective, Japan simply is a market to be exploited for selling goods manufactured in the United States, and barriers to imports are seen as a reproduction of protectionism. Likewise, Japanese supporters of national health insurance like to think of Japan's public health insurance program as a model for Americans. But there is also a dark side of Japanese medicine and clinical practice that has not been told.

Building on what is known about government and politics, including the bureaucracy over a period of time, the primary objective of this study is to disclose the embedded nature of regulation of medical devices and technologies in policy and institutional legacies. On this basis, Chapter 3 explores several background factors to medical technology regulation and discusses how they might bear on institutional change, the topic of the following chapter. Chapter 4 delves into the reform of the Pharmaceutical Affairs Law (PAL)—the most salient piece of legislation—and discusses why it was possible in 2005 and what the formal building blocks of medical technology regulation were intended to achieve. The analysis is limited to domestic factors. Chapter 5 takes up the question of how Japan responded to global pressures from the United States and the emerging single European market in 1987. Given the long-standing relationship between the US and Japan governments, the chapter also outlines a pattern of lobbying and interest group representation that emerged in the 1980s and remained fairly stable from the 1980s to the present. Chapter 6 examines the role of the Ministry of Health, Labor, and Welfare and the Pharmaceutical and Medical Devices Agency, which are in charge of medical device regulation and health care enforcement and implementation. In Chapter 7, I look into the role and the composition of the advisory committees that perform crucial advisory functions in the medical device field and bring in insights from regulatory science. Moreover, I explore how central controls over reimbursement may impact upon the "device lag." Chapter 8 scrutinizes clusters of government initiatives and government-sponsored operations to improve access to advanced medical technologies and clinical research infrastructure and to strengthen a weak medical-technological sector in Japan. Chapter 9 examines the realities of clinical medicine in Japan, with special reference to two remaining formal components of medical technology regulation, namely good clinical practice (GCP) and adverse event reporting (AER). The final chapter summarizes the major findings and offers concluding comments, leaving few puzzles unresolved.

Notes

1. Because of the important role of physicians in the use of medical devices and not just in the manufacture of a product, the terms *medical devices, medical products*, and *medical technology* are used interchangeably in this study.
2. This was historically the case in the United States until 1976, when medical device specific regulations were adopted. Prior to the establishment of the Single European Market through the Single European Act (SEA) in 1987,

most European countries regulated medical devices within the drug regulatory framework as well. An EU-wide regulatory framework for medical devices was established between 1990 and 1998, and it was established as a standalone framework separate from drugs.

3. Pammolli et al. depend heavily on the works of Alfred Kleinknecht, Kees van Montfort, and Eric Brouwer (2002), who developed proxies for studying technology in health care, but these proxies are limited for non-economic analyses.

4. Regulatory science is defined by the National Institutes of Health as "the development and use of the scientific knowledge, tools, standards, and approaches necessary for the assessment of medical product safety, efficacy, quality, potency and performance and the role of what is a specialized and interdisciplinary area of biomedical research that can generate new knowledge and tools for assessing experimental therapies, preventive therapies and diagnostics" (quoted by Yeo, 2010: 1).

5. Derrick Buddles from Stryker, a global orthopedics company, was chair of the MD&D, representing seventy-one medical device companies and about a quarter of the Japanese medical device and diagnostics market in 2007. See http://www.accj.or.jp (accessed 1/12/2008).

6. The ACCJ MD&D Subcommittee was renamed the American Medical Devices and Diagnostics Manufacturers' Association on April 1, 2009.

7. Cell and tissue engineering is defined as the regeneration of biological tissue through the use of cells, with the aid of supporting structured and/or biomolecules (European Commission, 2005).

8. Three examples will illustrate this point. First, Professor Teruo Okano, chair of the Institute for Advanced Bioengineering and Science is one of very few scholars working at the interface of medicine and bioengineering in Japan. (Yang et al., 2006a: 193–203; Yang et al., 2006b: 471–482; Yamato and Okano, 2004: 42–47); second, the Japanese achievements in cell engineering attracted the attention of British scholars (Williams, 2003: 1–59). David F. Williams wrote in the executive summary that the delegation found "more commonality than differences between the tissue engineering industry in Japan and the UK" (2003: 4). The third case is Professor Shinya Yamanaka from Kyoto University, who won a joint Nobel Prize in physiology for medicine in 2012.

9. HBD stands for harmonization-by-doing. See http://www.fda.gov.cdrh/internatinal/hdbpilot.htm (accessed 2007/03/30). This first meeting was four years in the making, but since the first meeting in January 2007, representatives from Japan and the United States have met on a regular basis, with the location rotating between Japan and the United States.

10. Before 2001, the Ministry of Health, Labor, and Welfare was named the Ministry of Health and Welfare (MHW).

11. Harmonization is an ambiguous concept. As used in this study, harmonization means bringing the various individual national regulatory policies and practices into line without any political intention of ever giving up one's own national practices. Convergence, in contrast, aims at a "single window" of global regulation with a simultaneous, explicit intention to reduce national regulation.

12. The six founding members of IMDRF—Australia, Brazil, Canada, EU, Japan, and the United States—were joined by China in March 2013 and Russia in August 2013. For more information, go to www.imdrf.org.

2

Knowledge, Analyses, and Experiences

Scholarship on Japan in three fields is extensive and indispensable for this monograph, as it provides valuable foundations for the arguments I develop. The objective of this chapter is to draw out the lessons from Japanese politics and policymaking—including the bureaucracy, health policy and health care system, and law and medicine—and to identify the descriptive characteristics of context conditions and salient structural elements and properties. The chapter concludes with a few fault lines associated with drawing the wrong lessons from Western experience and applying them to non-Western societies.

Scholarship on Japanese Politics, Policymaking, and the Bureaucracy

Scholarship on Japanese politics, policymaking, and bureaucracy examines the relationship between politicians, bureaucrats, and business over time. Scholars wrestle with key questions: who is leading in policymaking and controls the related processes? Who is being led, and how? Most studies favor the explanation of an "iron triangle" of corporations, bureaucratic ministries, and, to a lesser extent, political elites who have ruled Japan since World War II; yet there is by no means complete consensus on this argument (Kerbo and McKinstry, 1995: 173; Gary and Sone, 1993). Some studies argue that the leadership of the prime minister cannot be discarded entirely as leading policymaking occasionally (Hayao, 1993), while others point to the legislature (known as the Diet in Japan) as having a say in influencing legislation. But most agree that in the Japanese political economy, the Ministry of Finance and the Ministry of Economics, Trade, and Industry (METI) have historically been the most commanding (Hartcher, 1998).

Despite "Low Status," Gatekeeper and Arbiter

This literature rarely mentions the Ministry of Health,[1] but when it does, the ministry is classified as belonging to the "low status" ministries (Richardson, 1997). Hidehiko Kasahara (1999) gives a historical account of the Ministry of Health, which is also mentioned in the context of the contaminated blood scandal (e.g., Feldman, 1999), in scholarship on health policy and politics and law and medicine. John C. Campbell and Naoki Ikegami (1998), leading interpreters of the Japanese health care system and the health bureaucracy, inform about the enduring structural conditions, the compromising relationship of MHLW with the Japan Medical Association over time, and the macro-policy and micro-policy context in which payment policies are embedded and fees and prices finalized. The regulation of medical technologies is not their central concern (more on their interpretations later).

How to view the role of and actions by MHLW and the Pharmaceutical and Medical Device Agency (PMDA) in regulatory policymaking? I heavily draw on Campbell and Ikegami's work (1998), Suleiman (2003), Curtis (1999; 2002), Richardson (1997), and Schwartz and Pharr (2003). From this scholarship I can infer the key characteristics of the Japanese bureaucracy, which form the foundations into actions, possible motivations and bureaucratic behavior, and I can understand why officials do what they do and how they do it, concerning the review, registration, and approval of medical technologies for the Japanese market and different uses in health care. On advisory committees and their crucial role in policymaking, Frank J. Schwartz's interpretation of *shingikai,* or the politics of consultation, gives a taste of how the advisory councils and committees, which are established in the medical device field, may work. In reviewing an extensive literature on theories of interest group politics and policymaking in Japan, he underscores that interest groups are "*the* crucial institutions for explaining politics" in Japan, irrespective of a particular theoretical approach pursued by an author (Schwartz, 1998: ix, italics in original).[2] Adhering to a neo-pluralist approach, all authors provide descriptive characteristics of advisory committees and point out that the Japanese bureaucracy has been surprisingly proactive in the most important sectors of the economy in comparative perspective. Does the documented proactive governmental leadership role carry over to the medical technology sector, medicine, and medical research, and if not, why not? On advisory committees, are the properties of advisory committees in the medical device sector similar to those portrayed in this body of literature? Chapters 4, 5, and 6 will respond to these questions.

The Bureaucracy

John C. Campbell (1994: 114) describes a few characteristics of the bureaucracy in Japan: "[T]he tradition of bureaucratic dominance is stronger in Japan than in any other contemporary democracy." He stresses two further points. First, because of "a strong continuity with the prewar period . . . Japanese top officials are much more likely than their counterparts in the West to believe that they have the chief responsibility within their areas of jurisdiction for defining the national interest and determining major public policies" (Campbell, 1994: 116). This is in line with the evidence (provided below) that describes the MHLW, its image, and its self-perception, including its actions. Second, "Japanese ministries appear better able to maintain autonomy by controlling their own organizations" (Campbell, 1994: 117). And indeed they do, according to *Straitjacket Society* by Masao Miyamoto (1994), a medical doctor and insider to the health bureaucracy.

The only medical device-specific studies that I identified are two case studies written for and used at the Harvard Business School that address pressure group politics in the medical device sector. These cases vividly illustrate how American interests went about lobbying the relevant offices of MHLW, PMDA, and *Chuikyo*, the most important council for the public health insurance program in Japan, as well as other offices and bureaus. The first case traces the political conflicts between the US and Japanese governments over Japan's well-known protectionism, covering the period from the mid-1980s through 2000 (Watkins, 2004a). The second case explains why and how a major shift in the lobbying strategy of the US medical technology industry in Japan became necessary (Watkins, 2004b). The strategic questions were as follows: How can the US industry gain access to the Japanese market? What are the appropriate channels of communication and venues for interaction, apart from the bureaucracy? Which ones are promising? American business interests ranked contacts with Japanese by order of importance: first with politicians and government; second, with the regulatory agency; third, with surgeons; and finally, widely distributing information to the public.[3] These cases show an all-out campaign in action to gain access to the Japanese market.

Scholarship on Health Policy Studies and the Health-Care System in Japan

The literature on health policy and health-care reform in Japan is substantial and wide-ranging (Campbell and Ikegami, 2009: 265–287; Ikegami, 1999: 56–75; Ikegami, 2004: 26–35; Ikegami, 2009). It reveals the distinctive structural features of the health-care system and their strengths and weaknesses, leaving a trail of evidence in medical technology regulation, clinical research, and medical education, in addition to patient care and the quality of advanced treatments and procedures.

Achievements

Naoki Ikegami encapsulates the essence of the Japanese health care system as "an egalitarian system with universal coverage, social health insurance subsidized by taxes, excellent health indices, and no waiting list" (2007: 8–10). Japan provides universal coverage (see Table 2.1), low co-payments (starting with 10 percent in 1982, 20 percent in 1997, and later to 30 percent in 2003), and equitable access to quality care, including long-term care insurance in 2000 (Campbell and Ikegami, 2009).[4] National health expenditures are the lowest among the OECD countries, at 8 percent of GDP, but are expected to go up to 13.5 percent of GDP by 2035 (Kadonaga et al., 2008).

Doctor-Patient Relations

The doctor-patient relationship in Japan has been traditionally characterized by a firm hierarchy and submissive and non-empowered patients (Campbell and Ikegami, 2005; Campbell and Ikegami, 2009; Ikegami and Campbell 1999, 2004; Ikegami, 2009). Yet Naoki Ikegami reported at the *Leadership Dialogue for Stakeholders and Policy Leaders* in April 2007 on the changes in doctors' attitudes. Doctors have become more communicative and less arrogant when patients ask questions or ask for information. They no longer talk down to patients, as they used to do some forty years ago. They pay lip service to courtesy. But they are disinterested in how the system works (Ikegami, 2007: 8–10).

Table 2.1. Timeline of major health care reforms and policy measures, 1948–2006.

Year	Reform
1948	Enactment of the Medical Care Act
1961	Completion of the universal coverage of health insurance
1982	Health Services for the Elderly Act (financial redistribution for elderly care among insurers and public health services by municipal governments)
1985	First revision of the Medical Care Act (introduction of hospital bed control)
1992	Second revision of the Medical Care Act (introduction of hospitals with special functions supported by high technology and beds for the recovery of long-stay patients)
1997	Long-Term Care Insurance Act (took effect in April 2000)
1997	Third revision of the Medical Care Act (emphasis on informed consent, differentiation of regional tertiary hospitals) Fourth revision of the Medical Care Act (improved requirements of staffing and comfort)*
2002	Health Promotion Act (promotion of the people's health through improvement of the daily lifestyle)
2006	Structural Health Care Reform Act (fifth revision of the Medical Care Act, revision of the Health Services for the Elderly Act and other health insurance-related acts)

Source: Adapted from K. Tatara and E. Okamoto. Japan: Health system review. *Health Systems in Transition,* 2009: 11(5): 133.

*Note: In the literature on health systems, "amenity" refers to situations in which more comfort may be provided to a patient. For example, "amenity" may refer to the option for patients to be hospitalized in a two-bed room rather than a six-person room. German patients, for example, can purchase private health insurance for the privilege of having access to a one- or two-bed room and to the professor-surgeon rather than simply a less senior employed doctor. In addition, the nurse-patient ratio in Japanese hospitals is very low.

In the literature on health systems, "amenity" refers to situations in which more comfort may be provided to a patient. For example, "amenity" may refer to the option for patients to be hospitalized in a two-bed room rather than a six-person room. German patients, for example, can purchase private health insurance for the privilege of having access to a one- or two-bed room and to the professor-surgeon rather than simply a less senior employed doctor. In addition, the nurse-patient ratio in Japanese hospitals is very low.

Public Spending

The rise of health care expenditures in recent years in Japan is alleged to be due to four factors: advances in medical technology (estimated to make up 40 percent of the total increase); growing demand as a result of rising prosperity in Japan (26 percent); an aging population (18 percent); and new treatment patterns and a changing mix of diseases (16 percent, or the smallest portion of the total expected rise) (Kadonaga et al., 2008: 2–3). About 25 percent of Japan's total spending on health care goes to drugs and about 8 percent to medical devices (Wakao, 2007). The 8 percent only covers the medical products. I mention these data for two reasons: first, the industry has a strong interest in statistics that show low spending on medical technology over time and the contribution of medical technology to reduce overall health expenditures; second, 8 percent of public spending is "insignificant" in comparison to the costs of drugs and medical services. Quantitative data show the distribution of health expenditures, but they say little about the value of a medical device to an individual patient in need of a life-saving or life-sustaining medical device. For example, an insulin pump, which measures glucose levels every 5 minutes, 24 hours a day, is a life-saver for a diabetic. Or hip arthroplasty, usually known as "total hip replacement," is effective for elderly and middle-aged patients by increasing their well-being compared to the alternative of being seriously handicapped (and in the worst case, wheelchair-bound) for the rest of one's life. Finally, cataract surgery can remove a diseased lens and restore vision. All these procedures are included in the 8 percent mentioned above.

Given the economic stagnation in Japan that reigned during the 1990s, drugs and medical devices were caught between the government's preference to contain public spending in the health sector and an aging population's growing need of life-sustaining and life-assisting devices. This interpretation is convincing and on target. However, health policy experts do not agree; but they concede that Japan's traditional methods to control health care costs (such as increasing co-payments, insurance premiums, and tax subsidies combined with strict macro- and micro-managing efforts) may no longer be sufficient to close the ever-rising funding gap, and that health-care reform may have to coexist with solidarity- and market-based elements in order to keep health care affordable (Shibuya et al., 2011: 1265–1273; Ikegami et al., 2011: 1106–1115).

Ikegami and Campbell summarize the most constraining structural conditions in the Japanese health-care system, which are highly relevant for medical advances (2008: 107–113). Speaking to an uneven "medical axis of power," they argue that "the development of both specialists' and hospitals' organizations has been retarded" in Japan (Ikegami and Campbell, 2008: 108). Furthermore, they explain,

> Lacking such powerful constituencies, the Health Policy Bureau within the Ministry has tended to play second fiddle to the Health Insurance Bureau. However, private-practice physicians, who do not practice in hospitals, have been well organized under the Japan Medical Association (JMA). The JMA has managed to maintain its paramount position in organized medicine, despite the fact that the number of hospital-based physicians has increased to twice that of those who are office-based. As a result, resources have been prioritized to services provided in primary care settings, inhibiting the proliferation of high-tech, resource-intensive medicine. (2008: 108–109)

In the United States and Germany, for example, under comparable circumstances, professional specialists typically are the diffusers of medical technology into clinical practice and users of medical devices. Specialist physicians are key agents of medical innovation, clinical research, and clinical studies in these states. "[Physicians] made sure that no other professional group, government, or sickness fund payers are engaged in such activities" (Cohen and Hanf, 2004: 96–98). By contrast, in Japan in the past half-century, privately practicing physicians, organized in the Japan Medical Association (JMA), have enjoyed privileged access to the health bureaucracy, and they have called the shots over hospital-based physicians and scientifically oriented clinicians in third-tier hospitals (although the latter far outnumber the former).

The JMA has played a role in Japan that is not too different from the role professional organizations and professional politics have historically played in other countries. Concern for health care and better pay nationwide with no regional rate structure spurred the political activities of the JMA in the 1960s and 1970s (Steslicke, 1973: 236).[5] The fights of the medical profession in Japan were similar to the fights of the medical profession in the United States, Germany, France, the United Kingdom, and other Western countries. They targeted the maintenance of privileges, better pay, and professional autonomy. The socialization, professionalization, and specialization processes—internal to each medical profession—is specific to each country. The trajectory of the medical profession and the pathway to medical innovation in Japan stand out against the role of the medical profession in the United States and Europe (Abbot, 1988; Freddi and Björkman, 1989; Allsop and Mulcahy, 1996; Stevens, 2003 and 2006; Döhler 1992, 1997; Starr 1982; Freidson 1970a and 1970b). Depending on the country, the timing and sequence of events may have differed, but not the basic demands.[6] This general scenario contrasts enormously with the Japanese medical profession, the clannishness in recruitment of teaching positions based on personal relations, and the absence of a significant role for the community of specialists in professional politics in Japan.[7] At the time of writing, a few specialties had drafted guidelines on "best medical practice," but not all, which is significant for this study.

If the leaders of scientific medicine are not a driving force for making advanced medical technology available to patients, and if they are not the promoters of standards in medicine and medical specialties, and if specialists are not participating in writing the guidelines on "best medical practice" that doctors should follow when using and implanting a medical device in clinical practice, who takes their place? To whom does a technocratically inclined bureaucrat in the Ministry of Health turn for guidance in writing, for example, conflict-of-interest rules or prioritizing much-needed medical devices for fast-track approval? Who serves on advisory committees to MHLW or to *Chuikyo*, the decision-making body for the national health insurance program? Who provides the scientific knowledge: professional entrepreneurs interested in money and status, or scientifically inclined and research-oriented clinicians who are by no means uninterested in additional income?

Campbell and Ikegami (1998: 176–198) examined whether the continuous complaints about the bad quality of Japanese medicine by some Japanese (though mostly American) observers were justified. They looked at five quality problems in detail, as follows:

- Long waiting times and short consultation time, as summed up by the catch-phrase "wait for three hours, be seen for three minutes";
- Lack of information and accountability by physicians and within the health-care system generally;
- Run-down and understaffed hospitals that may not provide an adequate level of services and comfort for the patient;
- Low quantity and quality of medical research, particularly basic research;
- Poor quality of professional judgment in diagnosis and treatment.

They concluded that, overall, the criticism was valid. The problem listed last was the most "significant weak point in an evaluation of the overall quality of the Japanese health-care system" (1998: 176). Most deficiencies endure today, despite some initiatives.

Physician Users of Medical Devices

Japan allows primary-care physicians to prescribe and dispense drugs in outpatient care, an occurrence outlawed in other advanced societies. This raises thorny issues about incentives encouraging physicians to maximize their income, prestige, and dominance in professional affairs (Rodwin, 2011a: 161–183; 2011b: 184–203; 2011c; 1993). Do the same observations apply to physician users of medical devices? While medical devices are used in outpatient and inpatient care, physicians who use high-risk devices are typically employed staff with fixed incomes. If payoffs from the sale of medical devices are made, the extra income accrues primarily to hospital owners. Rodwin (2011a: 195) describes a scenario that is typical for the use of medical devices:

> Medical device manufacturers often bring their product to the surgeon at the time of surgery and sometimes prepare it for use and assist the physician. The hospital benefits because it does not have to stock supplies and keep inventory. The physician receives personal services and expert trouble shooting if problems arise. The practice creates loyalty since physicians need the seller's services. The seller obtains information on the physician's practice and needs and can recommend additional materials to a responsive purchaser. In this sort of relationship, which often involves multiple products, it is difficult for the physician to choose a lower cost option from another company. (Rodwin, 2011a: 195)

Providing on-site assistance to physicians reinforces brand loyalty and seems to be an integral part of doing business in Japan, as in the United States and elsewhere. In Japan, it also happens because "skilled nursing staff . . . is not often available in Japan making on-site expertise indispensable" (MTLF, 2007: 19). Yet this story leaves out one loophole: the fee-for-service reimbursement for surgery under the Japanese DPC-based hospital compensation system[8] leaves sufficient incentives for hospital doctors to do more than is "medically necessary." Other advanced societies have eliminated fee-for-service reimbursement from hospital compensation over the years in order to contain ever-rising hospital costs. There is no empirical study on the prevalence of such behavior in Japan. Nevertheless, a few interviewees insinuated that more treatments and procedures might be done than are "medically necessary" (Interview #43; Interview #16; Interview #36). In sum, with the exception of Rodwin (1993; 2011a; 2011b and 2011c), Campbell and Ikegami (1998), and Ikegami and Campbell (2008), authors writing on health-care reform in Japan do not address the implications of the reforms for the utilization of medical devices in therapies.

The quotes from Ikegami (2008) below focus on the most salient characteristics of the delivery of health care and the behavior and attitudes of Japanese physicians. These quotes describe the structural conditions where medical devices are used, post-market surveillance carried out, and medical-technological innovations and treatment advances performed. These contextual conditions are so fundamental to this study that I quote at length from this source, even though the study does not focus on clinical practice per se. These statements help one understand how regulatory processes of medical devices functioning at the macro- and micro-levels of the political and the health-care system are structured, and why they delay or block the approval of innovative medical devices in Japan. It also becomes clear why Dr. Minami's personal experience (discussed in Chapter 1) is representative of a structural pattern of clinical practice and training in Japan rather than the experience of one individual.

> The hierarchical and closed structure of physicians retarded the development of professional specialist organizations. Since career advancement depended on the evaluation by their professors, young physicians tended to focus more on research than on acquiring clinical skills. Their objective lay in obtaining the research degree of Doctor of Medical Science, which came to be regarded as a mark of professional competence by the public because there was no formal system of certification as specialists. Most physicians went into private practice in midlife, upon which they would lose access to hospital facilities. Thus, physicians in clinics usually focused on primary care. (Ikegami, 2008: 2).

> The biomedical healthcare system is characterized by the following features . . . First is the lack of standardization and quality control. Most hospital physicians have been appointed to their positions within the closed network of hospitals affiliated with the university clinical department. Although two-thirds of the physicians are now certified as specialists, only about half have undergone a formal training postgraduate training process and the rest have been grandfathered in based on their experience. . . . Second is the lack of differentiation between generalists and specialists, and between acute care and long-term care (LTC) facilities. As noted, certification

as a specialist has been slow to develop. Physicians may profess and practice in any speciality they may choose, while patients can directly access any physician they wish, including those in tertiary care. . . . Third is the high level of hospital beds at 14.3 per one thousand population, while the staffing level of nurses remains low at one nurse for twenty-two inpatients. These actors, together with the lack of differentiation between acute care and LTC, have contributed to the long average length of stay, 36 days (if LTC hospital beds are excluded, it would still be 20 days. (Ikegami , 2008: 2–3).

The central message is clear: without specialization, there is no innovation or medical progress. Without specialization, there are no advanced treatments or clinical trials.

Medical Training

Japanese experts agree that Japan lacks sizeable, competent, and extensive resources and capabilities for the conduct of clinical research, despite the fact that eighty medical schools have existed since 1980 (Tatara and Okamoto, 2009: 90). The clinical research infrastructure is weak; for decades, it has been neglected and ignored by politicians and bureaucratic policymakers alike. Tatara and Okamoto note that "Postgraduate medical training has been poorly developed in Japan" (2009: 93), and that "Contrary to the belief that Japan has a widespread advanced computer technology, IT has not been well developed in health care" (2009: 88). Two sources (Interview #32 and Interview #12) described Japanese physicians as combining professional and entrepreneurial features in such ways that a deep split between scientific medicine and primary-care physicians has existed for decades, which in turn also has exerted negative effects on medical innovation and clinical research. Discharging patients too early often results in repeat admissions, as is reported for the United States, and keeping them for too long, as is the case of Japan, results from a combination of factors: the existing health-care infrastructure, availability of trained nursing staff, and the ways hospitals are compensated for providing hospital care. Ikegami explains, "LTC (long-term care) beds are covered by health insurance and functioning as *de facto* nursing homes" (2008: 3). Social services were not developed early in Japan; the "medicalization of LTC" (2008: 2) was not matched with putting resources into building nursing home facilities. Table 2.2 below shows the outlier status of Japan in terms of hospital days and hospital beds per one thousand people, including the low number of inspectors who monitor the implementation of drug and medical device regulation in comparison to Western countries.[9]

Table 2.2. Select hospital data.

Country	Average days in hospital	Doctors per 1,000 population	Hospital beds per 1,000 population	Number of inspectors
Japan	36.3	3.0	14.2	197
US	6.5	2.4	3.3	2,200
Germany	10.4	3.4	8.6	1,100
France	13.4	3.4	7.5	900
UK	7.2	2.3	4.0	693

Source: ACCJ Journal, November 2007, Vol. 44(1): 21.

Finally, Koichi Kawabuchi reports on research on elderly patients with hip fracture, with a focus on finding out the link between the length of stay (LOS) and walking ability (2006: 1589–1596). The research differentiated between LOS that included days at transferred hospitals and cost performance. Finally, the author compared the Japanese procedure and schedules with data from the United Kingdom and the United States:

> We found a positive relationship between LOS and walking ability. LOS required to gain final walking ability was shorter when a single hospital completed the procedure. Japan had more than 3 times longer LOS than the other two countries, due to more variety of procedures and longer interval between steps. (Kawabuchi, 2006: 1589–1596)

Why empirical data are so scarce is also deeply rooted in social science traditions in Japan. First, Yamada et al. (2006) explain that "empirical research in Japan is theoretically and economically inferior to that of the United States, especially at the micro-level of policy-oriented research" (2006: 23).[10] They give three reasons: first, government-initiated research data are not released to the public or researchers and universities, unlike in most cases in American or European practice; second, few doctors in Japan are involved in clinical research; and third, unlike pharmaeconomics in the United States and Europe, "Japan does not apply health economic analysis to clinical testing in the approval of new medicines" (Yamada et al., 2006: 23). In 2004, Japan took modest steps to introduce a health technology assessment capability (HTA) (Oliver, 2003; Oliver et al., 2004). Adam Oliver argues that "the fee-for-service and strict price regulation that characterizes the system of health care financing in Japan is not conducive to this form of analysis" (2003: 197–204).

While this scholarship provides much circumstantial evidence, we need to move toward more specific questions concerning medical technologies. Why is there little or no research on medical devices, product unavailability, and utilization? Why are the data so limited? And finally, why do the Japanese lag in access to innovative medical technologies and advanced treatments in Japan in comparison to patients in Europe or the United States? To repeat, on average, Japanese patients have access to advanced therapies and medical and surgical procedures between three to six years later than in other advanced industrialized nations (Chapter 2). Surgeons in the United States and Europe use the fifth or sixth generation of pacemakers, while cardiologists in Japan can only use third-generation pacemakers due to cost-containment policies, according to Dr. Minami. The Japanese government's preference for macro-managing total health expenditures and micro-managing physician behavior through fee schedules, price controls, and other restrictive measures is widely documented. These constraints ring true, despite different interpretations by scholars about cause and effect of rising health expenditure and cost-containment policies.

Standards

A 2009 official publication provides information on the organization, financing, regulation, planning, and resources of the health-care system in Japan (Tatara and Okamoto, 2009). It discusses at length the regulation of pharmaceuticals, the evaluation of new drug applications, and the government's supervision of the pharmaceutical industry over manufacturing, clinical trials, and post-marketing surveillance (Tatara and Okamoto, 2009: 74). It even mentions that eight divisions of the Ministry of Health draft and write the rules on the manufacturing of drugs, known as good manufacturing practice (GMP), good clinical practice (GCP), and good post-marketing study practice (PMS). This official publication does not waste a word explaining that the same or similar rules on GMP, GCP, and GMP apply to the medical device side, the use of medical devices, and the medical technology industry as well as clinical trials with medical devices or *ex post* marketing controls. The rules for clinical trials of medical devices were explained to be "almost identical with those for pharmaceuticals" (Mitsumori, 2006a; 2006b).

By way of summary, the aim of this extensive review of a body of literature on health policy and the health-care system was to learn about the contextual conditions and causal factors that might contribute to explaining the device "lag." These structural conditions in health and clinical practice and related stumbling blocks are instrumental in constraining the modernization of the regulatory structure; influencing the reimbursement scheme of prescription drugs and medical devices under the Japanese public health protection scheme; shaping the biannual revisions of the reimbursement scheme to contain costs within a macro-policy and micro-management context; and, finally, they reveal a noteworthy "asymmetrical axis of power." No other source of information could provide a better foundation to begin this study.

Scholarship on Medicine and Law

How do legal scholars respond to issues and problems that arise from the medical profession, medicine, clinical practice, and crises in health? For example, these issues concern conflict-of-interest issues in physician-patient relations and in the prescribing and dispensing behavior of doctors, including receiving gifts and payments from the industry (Rodwin, 1993, 2011a, 2011b; Rodwin 2011c; Rodwin and Okamoto, 2000). The very low reporting of adverse events associated with inappropriate prescription and dispensation of drugs or medical devices by Japanese physicians is documented (discussed later) and is of particular relevance. Legal research also studies accreditation, certification, and continuing medical education in Japan. Several authors (Rodwin, 1993; Rodwin and Okamoto, 2000; Leflar, 2007 and 2009; and Nomi, 1999)[11] investigate quality assurance, utilization review, and oversight as well as Japanese tort law, patient safety issues, and medical errors. Luke Nottage analyzed product liability law (2004, 2005). Eric A. Feldman studied organ transplants and patients' rights and movements (1994, 1997, 2000). In his study on the HIV-contaminated blood scandal, Feldman (1999) contends that a new era in tort law has opened as a result of this scandal in the 1990s. He gives four causes for this alleged change: a growing awareness of the Japanese public and society at large, the erosion of the Japanese people's trust in their physicians, media attention to these matters, and an increasing number of attorneys who now can take up medical litigation cases (Japan Public Health Association, 2007: 50–51).

Norio Higuchi, professor of law at the University of Tokyo's Law School, and his research team and previous doctoral students, such as Dr. Tomoko Mise and Dr. Chiaki Sato, who has been working on medical devices since 2011, are at the forefront of related research, extensively scrutinizing conflict-of-interest issues primarily associated with prescribing and dispensing of drugs but also with the regulation of medicine, medical law, and medical information (Higuchi, 2005, 2007a, 2007b, 2007c, and 2007d). A trusted adviser to Japanese officials in the Ministry of Health, he also closely collaborates with a few practicing lawyers who are well-known experts in medical law and drug law, such as Tatsuo Kuroyanagi (2002 and 2005; Kuroyanagi et al. 2004, 2005) and academics like Robert B. Leflar and Futoshi Iwata (2006). Norio Higuchi and all his collaborators, senior and junior alike, were valuable resource persons for this project.

In addition, Yutaka Tejima (1993) examines tort law, compensation, and medical malpractice, as well as adverse events resulting from drugs. Kazue Nakajima et al. (2001: 1632) examined closely the rise of medical malpractice claims and the size of indemnity payments over the last thirty years, which still are considerably lower than in the United States. Japanese and American legal scholars report that medical professionals are reluctant to serve as experts in medical malpractice litigation. For example, Sakamoto et al. (2002) compare Japanese practices with those in France and Germany. They describe the situation as follows:

> In Japan, in contrast to European countries, such as France and Germany, there is insufficient cooperation in medical malpractice litigation by medical experts . . . There are a small number of practitioners in Japan who undertake the role of medical expert but not from a neutral standpoint. A formal system would serve to dilute the power of dishonest practitioners . . . Most medical professionals refuse the request of the courts to assist with the use of medical knowledge . . . The percentage of cases making use of experts over the last 10 years was 22.5%, with regional variations between 33.3% highest and 3.4% the lowest when the court had not engaged any lawyer at all. (Sakamoto et al., 2002: 201).

Finally, for cultural reasons, Japanese patients are more reluctant to give their informed consent than their European and American counterparts (Annas and Miller, 1994).

By way of summary, from this legal scholarship we can infer a few striking observations pertinent to this study on medical technology regulation. First, existing law restrains the opportunities for change and even creates barriers with serious implications for the regulation of medical devices and the medical device sector in general. Second, the concept of privacy in Japan differs from that prevailing in Western societies and, according to Norio Higuchi (2007c, 2007d), leads to excessive regulation of medical information. Third, the Japanese legal order overwhelmingly relies on criminal law in malpractice litigation in contrast to Western countries; civil law malpractice litigation is infrequent (Leflar, 2009; Leflar and Iwata, 2006, 2005). Reviewers of medical devices for market approval are personally held responsible for their decisions. Fourth, Japanese people turn to prosecutors and the police when they feel they are the victims of medical errors. This seems to be the only option in light of the absence of professional accountability mechanisms, a functioning peer review system, and professional discipline structures. Finally, hospital accreditation is not mandatory. These factors, taken together, hardly nurture a culture of professional responsibility, transparency, and accountability, nor do they foster support for patient rights.

MHLW and Conflicts of Interest

In January 2008, MHLW officials were working with an advisory group to develop rules on conflicts of interest in the drug area.[12] I was privileged to attend one of the closed meetings, hoping to learn whether this work eventually would apply to medical technologies. I learned from the officials in charge of medical devices that "whatever rules are now on the books are sufficient to handle any eventualities of conflicts of interest with medical devices" (Interview #34; Interview #47). Obviously, this is a matter of interpretation.

How to explain this silence on medical devices? A first explanation interprets the integration of medical device regulation into the drug regulatory framework as an illustration of a widespread belief and a widely shared assumption that rules for drugs automatically apply to medical devices without qualification. This belief and related assumptions are misguided. But I encountered evidence of such cognitive dissonance throughout this study. Second, MHLW could have added medical devices to its work on drugs but chose not to. Why? From the literature on the bureaucracy and health policy analysis I infer two observations: first, the MHLW continues to be under the spell of the JMA and its political allies; and second, the JMA is by no means ceding political space to MHLW to write rules on conflicts of interest that would affect the physician-members of the JMA.

This is not to say that there are no rules of ethics that apply to Japanese physicians. A first code was adopted in 1951 consisting of 150 words. It stated six principles, among them, "The physician will not engage in medical activities for profit-making motives" (Rodwin,

2011a: 172–173). It is clear that the code did not address conflict-of-interest issues as they are discussed today in the United States and in other Western nations. Nor were these addressed in a seventeen-page code published in 2002. In 2003, JMA was working again on a new code but excluded conflict-of-interest issues (Interview #58; Interview #11). Instead, according to Rodwin, "[T]he JMA has championed the prohibition of investor-owned hospitals and portrayed physician-owned hospitals as the not-for-profit alternative. That allowed physicians free rein as medical entrepreneurs" (2011a: 172–173).

The notion of self-regulation by professional groups, as generally understood in the West, is underdeveloped in Japan. The Japanese medical profession meets two of three attributes that, according to Eliot Freidson (1970a; 1970b), characterize a profession: *control* over clinical practice, *autonomy* (the quality or state of being independent, free, and self-directing), and *a code of ethics* (Rodwin, 2011a: 199–201). While rudimentary ground rules for conflicts of interest in drug manufacturer-physician relations were being rewritten in 2008, none was expected to address the users of medical devices (Interview #56).

Stakeholder groups—that is, doctors, industry, and regulators—do not talk to each other, which certainly does not secure ethical behavior, and the opposite may be true (Rodwin, 2011a: 194–199). One source (Interview #28) insisted on a favorite Japanese behavior pattern of not doing anything until something bad happens. Then there is reaction, perhaps overreaction, and the pendulum swings back from one extreme to another. If anybody can act to remedy this problem, it would have to be the government (Interview #28). The government can monitor, but it chooses not to. For example, JMA received ten million dollars annually to fund investigators to explore orphan drugs and orphan medical devices. Orphan drugs and orphan medical devices are products that have been developed for rare diseases and conditions and have been granted legal status. The disclosure of financial interests was not monitored (Interview #28). The Orphan Drug Act in the United States specifically addresses drugs and medical devices separately, while the existing provisions in Japan and the European Union primarily refer to drugs only and not to medical devices. In the final analysis, the question is raised whether anybody—the government, industry, or clinicians, including the JMA—really has an interest in writing strict rules on conflict-of-interest issues. Thus far, a political will to write stricter rules on conflict of interest has existed only for drugs.

Decision-Maker and Judge

How did legal scholarship respond to the HIV and blood scandal in Japan in the mid-1990s? Interested in how health crises are handled, Feldman (1999) identified four salient features reflecting the influence of political culture: (i) a foreign (US) source of a domestic crisis; (ii) a preference for blaming individuals rather than the health bureaucracy (MHLW); (iii) a claim that Japanese conflicts are "unique" and of no interest to outsiders; and finally (iv) lessons Japanese policymakers did not learn. Unlike most Western countries (Feldman and Bayer, 1999), Japan did not create independent commissions to investigate the causes and consequences of the blood scandal. The same Ministry of Health, whose officials made wrong decisions in responding to the crisis, was in charge of investigating the scandal.[13] This sounds all too familiar, with what the mass media reported on various health-care crises.[14] They reported on unavailable cancer treatments in Japan (until very recently), the delay in making silicon breast implants available (which may have been beneficial to Japanese women), and adverse events related to drugs and underperforming medical products, as well as medical errors.

Emerging Case Law

With an increased use of medical technologies in medical practice, more litigation involving medical devices can be expected. The legal umbrella is tort law, as it is for medicine, apparatuses, and malpractice. Case law on the safety of medicine exists, but case law on medical devices is practically nonexistent in Japan, explained Tatsuo Kuroyanagi, senior partner with law firm Kaneko and Iwamatsu in Tokyo, and Shinichi Murata, a junior lawyer. According to them, only a handful of practicing lawyers are knowledgeable in matters of medicine and law. On medical devices, an effective lawyer must also be knowledgeable in intellectual property rights to handle medical device-related cases. On the court's side, they estimated that fewer than five judges in all may be competent to rule on medical device-related cases. By January 2008, three court rulings had been adjudicated that genuinely illustrate that case law on medical devices is beginning to evolve—an indication of the limited awareness in Japan of medical devices used in health care.

Drawing the Wrong Conclusions from Western Experience

Medical professionals are the most dynamic forces to bring modern medical technologies to patient care by adopting and using them in clinical practice and diffusing them throughout the delivery system of medical services (Cohen and Hanf, 2003; Battista et al., 1994). Internships in medicine were only mandated in 2004 in Japan; uniform curricula for specialty training were required around the same time, and continuing education in medicine was only mandated in 2005.

Medical specialization and internships in the West have been an integral part of medical education in the United States and Europe since the early twentieth century, with the medical profession asserting itself in writing the curriculum for medical specialty training, internships, and accreditation. In contrast, sub-specialization and what often appears as sub-sub-specialization are post-1945 phenomena in the United States and European countries alike. By the same token, the requirements for continued medical education (CME) to maintain medical knowledge and keep up with change in health care were formalized and institutionalized in the United States in the 1970s and further formalized in multiple but different modes in subsequent decades. The medical professions in various European countries responded several years later. Today, CME is on the professional books in one form or another in most European countries (Mladovsky et al., 2009: 1–12). However, it is a big business, and it raises numerous conflict-of-interest issues in the United States and Europe (Steinbrook, 2009).

On January 28, 2013, I spoke with Hideo Tsukamoto, former executive director of the Japan Federation of Medical Devices Association (JFMDA) for twenty years until 2007; he had published a short history in Japanese that documents the increasing involvement of JFMDA in international standard setting and regulatory affairs (Tsukamoto, 1999a, 1999b). A timeline running from the early 1990s to the present clearly indicated the rising internationalization of medical device regulatory affairs in Japan via the participation of Japanese officials and experts in the meetings of the technical committees of the International Standards Organization (ISO/TC), various joint EU-FDA initiatives, and finally Japan's participation in the work of the Global Harmonization Task Force (GHTF), a joint forum for regulators and industry, which ended in 2011. It was replaced by the International Medical Device Regulatory Forum (IMDRF). As a founding member of the GHTF, Japan continues to be an active participant in the IMDRF. During this twenty-year period, the Global Medical Device Conference, an industry-only forum, often met parallel to the GHTF. The activities pursued by the GHTF and the IMDRF suggest that salient national regulatory issues some twenty years ago have become increasingly transnational and international regulatory issues that trickle down to domestic settings through multilevel venues (Wessel and Wouters, 2008). The Japanese case well illustrates this increasing interdependence and internationalization of regulatory affairs.

By way of summary, the knowledge, analyses, and experiences offered by American and Japanese academics form valuable foundations into the investigation of the regulation of medical technologies and provide a precious background for this study. These insights into different facets of government, law and medicine, and health policy research in Japan, taken together, plausibly justify a challenge to the conventional wisdom of why Japan suffers from "device lag" and, instead, offer alternative or complementary interpretations and explanation of the "device lag." According to the conventional wisdom, the persistent fault line underlying the huge paradoxes encountered in the medical technology sector in Japan is primarily due to the engrained bureaucratic traditions in rule-making and rule application, bureaucratic rigidities, and a legalistic and formalistic administrative culture, including a lack of governmental vision and leadership in advancing medicine in Japan and strengthening the medical technology sector. These arguments were advanced by Japanese free-market supporters of deregulation, privatization, and liberalization as much as by representatives of US-based device makers, a few scholars, and journalists.

These factors, no doubt, contribute to why the "device lag" exists and why a good many medical technologies in Japan are unavailable. These explanations, however, are only first-order explanations. Second-order explanations are more deeply rooted. Chief among them are the backwardness of Japanese medicine and its specialties and sub-specialties, an absence of opinion leaders driving medical innovations (with the notable exception of isolated individuals and institutions), the absence of a scientific medical community internalizing and practicing the norms of excellence, and the lack of openness and transparency of clinical research results among peers. And last but not least, the status quo of clinical medicine and clinical infrastructures is untenable. In the final analysis, neither the bureaucracy nor the medical profession or the scientific communities are agents of change; more appropriately, they are status quo agents primarily. This is not to say that the reform of medical device regulation and the current promotion of clinical and medical capabilities are not also heavily colliding with a tradition that puts rigid rule-making and law and public administration over common sense, pragmatism, and open public discourse. Moreover, the way the legal medical device framework was framed and constructed in Japan fundamentally clashes with the true nature of most sophisticated medical technologies, and high-risk implants in particular. As previously stated, drugs and the majority of medical devices are entirely different products that contribute different inputs to health outcomes. Each product category follows a different innovative path prior to ever reaching the market. Yet there is only one policy frame, the Pharmaceutical Affairs Law (PAL). It is a one-size-fits-all umbrella of rules, norms, and procedures applicable to both product categories, notwithstanding a few isolated medical device-specific rules, standards, and review guidelines. This has been the status quo since 2005. However, a new actor constellation will appear that may create new political and bureaucratic dynamics after the revision of PAL, which will come into effect in September 2014.

Notes

1. The Ministry of Health was restructured in 2002 and became the Ministry of Health, Labor, and Welfare (MHLW). For simplicity's sake, I refer to MHLW or the Ministry of Health (MOH).
2. Schwartz summarizes the key idea of the authors on the importance of institutions in Japan: "Whatever their differences, every school has acknowledged the role of *shingikai*, Japan's consultative councils." Johnson: "To the extent that laws are scrutinized and discussed at all in Japan by persons outside the bureaucracy, it is done in the councils." Pempel: Advisory bodies "have become major organizational tools in overall policy formation." Muramatsu and Krauss: "There are constant attempts to coordinate and structure the keen intra- and intersectoral competition. The use of *shingikai* to hammer out acceptable policy solutions among competing interests is one such coordinative device." Campbell: "Consensus within the policy community is virtually a prerequisite for an idea to be taken seriously by others. Such a consensus is usually embodied in the formal report by the legally established advisory committee for that policy area." Kumo: "*Shingikai* are the most representative form of network organizations connecting industrial, political, mass media, and academic spheres to one another." (Schwartz, 1998: 40–47.)
3. The publication of the so-called Bain study is said to have been instrumental in this campaign.
4. Naoki Ikegami, in a lecture entitled "Containing Healthcare Expenditures in Japan" on November 5, 1999, at the Mailman School of Public Health, Columbia University, offered his interpretation of the ongoing health-care reform.
5. Steslicke talks about two items of concern to the JMA: the operation of the health insurance system and the right of doctors to prescribe and sell medicine.
6. The literature on medical specialization in comparative perspective is abundant but selectively referenced in this chapter.

7.   The Royal Academy of Engineering Mission to Japan under the mission leader Professor David F. Williams, in its examination of how Japan could improve its capacities in the field of tissue engineering, recommends addressing the lack of qualified personnel, relaxing the hierarchy model within universities, enhancing entrepreneurship within universities, making suitable facilities available, and improving access to funding and a clear regulatory route to markets.

8.   DPC stands for diagnostic-procedure combination, while DRGs stand for diagnostic-related groups. DRG-based payments to hospitals are used in Europe and the United States. A major difference between the two hospital payment systems is that the DPC retains a fee-for-service element for a number of items, including surgical procedures benefiting either the hospital or the operating surgeon, while the DRG-based reimbursement does not.

9.   These data are not the best, but they are the only ones available that shed light on how many inspectors are available to monitor what goes on at the hospital management end. The OECD and the WHO have superior databases, but they do not include inspections.

10. The authors examine how Japan measures up to eight criteria set by the World Health Organization.

11. Starting with the history of Japanese law, Nomi then goes on to discuss a wide range of the sources of law (the rule of law, the Constitution, statute law, delegation legislation, international treaties, judge-made law, circulars, administrative guidance, local regulations, customary law, and scholarly opinion) and covers all aspects of Japanese law. These illustrations can (but need not) be sources of law applicable to medical technology regulation.

12. The minutes of the meeting were available in March 2008 from http://wwwhaisin.mhlw.go.jp/mhlw/C/?c=124579.

13. A major reorganization of the Ministry of Health followed considerably later.

14. A search of the archives of www.asahi.cm/english/ for the years 2007 and 2008 was done; and a Nikei Premium-English/Archive Search covering the period from 1990 to 2008 was run. With the exception of specific periods, the yield on medical device-specific articles was modest.

3

Medical Technology Regulation

This chapter addresses how the intentions of the Pharmaceutical Affairs Law (PAL) are translated into action and how PAL is experienced by officials and business. PAL is embedded in a path-dependent institutional and organizational environment, but it also introduces novel elements of policy and law. The chapter is divided into two parts. The first begins by tracing the historical trajectory of the regulation, and how and why it was possible to enact the Pharmaceutical Affairs Law (PAL) in 2005, despite persistent structural constraints in Japan. To do so, the chapter identifies the main drivers of change and then explores the political circumstances that brought about change. After a brief sketch of the political conditions, public opinion, and a widespread distrust toward physicians, the chapter also lays out the objectives of the PAL and the formal building blocks of medical device regulation. In the second section, I offer several narratives and anecdotes, based on interviews, to shed light on the enforcement and implementation *de jure* and *de facto*. In this context, it will become clear how and why medical technology regulation in Japan differs from that in the United States and the EU.

A Cross-National Perspective

The emergence of the regulatory framework of medical devices in Japan over the last twenty years occurred in political circumstances that are dramatically different from those in the United States and the European Union. In the United States, the FDA-based regulatory framework evolved in a political climate of democratic changes in political and executive leadership within a political and legal system of checks and balances for over a hundred years, starting shortly after the turn of the twentieth century (Carpenter, 2010). By contrast to the centralized decision-making structure in the United States, the

EU medical device regulatory framework emerged as part of market-creating measures of the single European market after 1987, through a shift in regulatory powers over competition and commercial policies from the member states to EU institutions. The descriptive characteristics of the EU-wide regulatory regime are as follows: it is a transnational and multilevel stand-alone framework for medical devices separate from drugs; it combines centralized and decentralized decision-making processes with highly decentralized enforcement and implementation in the EU member states (Altenstetter, 2008, 2012, and 2013).

By contrast, in Japan the Liberal Democratic Party (LDP) was in power for some fifty years, starting in 1955; it introduced the major health-care programs in the 1950s and successively extended coverage to different population groups. Universal coverage was achieved in 1961. In the subsequent decades, the LDP was busy amending the same programs by reducing the differences in benefits among the Japanese as a result of legislation aimed at distinct population groups (Ikegami and Campbell, 2008). The LDP also oversaw major administrative reforms from the 1970s to the present, with a leading role ceded to a *proactive civil service* (Pempel and Muramatsu, 1995; Pempel, 1992). The uninterrupted rule of the governing party—described as a "one-party dominant system" (Tanabe, 1997) or "the circulating cast of elite leadership" (Otake, 2000: 291–310)—ended in 2007 when the LDP lost control over the second chamber. The LDP was entirely wiped from its leadership position in August 2009 when Yukio Hatoyama led the Democratic Party to a landmark victory in elections. However, in May 2010, after less than a year in office, he resigned as prime minister under considerable pressure from the Japanese public for breaking a campaign promise to move the US military base in Okinawa further north. He was succeeded by Prime Minister Naoto Kan of the Democratic Party of Japan (DPJ) in 2012, who was followed by Prime Minister Abe (LDP) in 2013.

The LDP oversaw the enactment of PAL in 2002 and its radical revamping in 2005, placing numerous barriers to the approval and diffusion of medical technologies in Japan (the Pharmaceutical Affairs Law, 2005; 2005–2006; 2005/07). Between 2005 and the beginning of 2014 PAL has been the most significant piece of legislation for medical devices, but also a highly ambivalent one. The health bureaucracy heavily borrowed from the US FDA and the EU, which squarely falls in line with a characterization of lawmaking and policymaking in Japan, often cited by scholars such as Tanabe (1997: 117), in which "imitation plays a more important role than innovation." The bureaucracy drafted a bill largely integrating the international Summary Technical Document (STED) into a domestic piece of legislation. Japan, the European Union, the United States of America, Australia, and Canada, through their cooperation in the GHTF, agreed upon STED as a global model of harmonization in the field of medical devices. The Japanese legislature approved the draft without major debate. The bureaucracy was also busy issuing an array of enforcement orders and ministerial ordinances on PAL (in fact, a total of 150 new regulation and guidance documents had to be implemented by April 1, 2005) (USITC, 2007: 6–12). Finally, the LDP also oversaw the creation of the Pharmaceutical and Medical Device Agency (PMDA) in 2004 (PMDA on the Internet, 2005 and 2006).

I was interested in finding out why these changes were made. Did PAL in 2005 and the creation of the PMDA the previous year come about as a result of external pressures, were they internally driven, or both? Do these changes represent a novel form of institutional change that was not encountered in the past? How unique are they? On the basis of much documented evidence there cannot be any doubt that the most important external stimuli, prompting the legislative and organizational changes, came from outside Japan. The same practices of adapting foreign ideas from the West and the same "mechanism of institutional reconstruction" were at work. This was entirely in line with a long-established pattern of institutional change since the nineteenth century. In Muramatsu and Krauss's view (1996: 210), "imitation and innovation" go hand in hand, but "tradition was recast for the purpose of the organization, rather than reshaping the Western model to fit Japanese traditions" (1996: 219). After 1945, these authors found "a mixture of foreign emulation and domestic continuity" (Muramatsu and Krauss, 1996: 220).

The attitudes of Japanese patients carry considerable weight in health care and medical innovation. Japanese patients are said to be distrustful and reluctant to enroll in clinical trials, which, in turn, negatively impacts upon clinical research and medical innovation. The Japanese are also said to be disinclined to allow the release or use of personal health information (Interview #4; Interview #18; Interview #20; Interview #22; Interview #32; Interview #35; Interview #36; Interview #48; Interview #51; and Interview #52). According to these informants, the Japanese are extremely risk-averse. Legal scholarship adds weight to this assessment (Higuchi, 2007c, 2007d). Moreover, "Japanese patients have very little access to information about healthcare opportunities or even some treatments available inside Japan" said Mr. Plunkett, as quoted by Alex Wood (2009; also Leflar, 1996).

Speaking for the med-tech industry, Dr. Huimin Wang was quoted by the same source as having said, "It's even worse for us. For medical devices, the issue is harder for the public to understand. It's more technological."[1] A health official, close to the then Safety Division (Interview #37) explained, "Japanese people expect the government to implement a policy of zero risk in regard to drugs, medical devices and food. But when something happens, they blame the government." Reference to an alleged "blaming culture" was a constant during the interviews.

In a second interview on January 24, 2008, the same official (Interview #53) explained that if Japanese patients want new and advanced treatments and are willing to pay for them, they must also learn to accept the results of clinical tests and treatments. If an advanced treatment is approved by the authority and an adverse event with a medical device (a near miss or fatal incident) occurs afterward, then patients begin to worry about the side effects and refuse to accept the earlier promises of clinical results. Japanese people can be quite "unforgiving and intolerant," accusing the government and the Ministry of Health of wrong-doing.

According to an industry insider who echoed similar sentiments (Interview #23), there is a real problem. Regulation is a job for regulators, but part of the problem is also the general public. Japanese people feel that the government must resolve everything, including strict regulation (Interview #23). But why should the government do it? Why not ask for better self-regulation by the industry? In his view, the Japanese people distrust the industry, hence they think that government must regulate. The Japanese people get the government they voted for (Interview #23). In theory, the government could provide better leadership for medical technologies, but in reality, the people need to vote for better government first (Interview #23).

Since the Japanese lack confidence in doctors and trust in clinical decision-making, the question arises: what are the root causes of such lack of confidence in doctors and health care and their distrust in general and toward medical technology and clinical research in particular? What is known about trust or distrust of Japanese people vis-à-vis government and politics? Drawing on data from cross-national research (Pharr, 2000: 173–201), the Japanese (27 percent) ranked low in trust in politics, next to Italians with 22 percent. The rankings for other states include the United States (31 percent), Britain (45 percent), Germany (69 percent), the Netherlands (58 percent), and Austria (71 percent).

Observers of Japanese politics and society come up with three different interpretations explaining why the Japanese lack confidence and are distrustful. Peter Katzenstein (2000: 202–228) concludes "Japan has not seen political confidence plummet from high levels . . . By most anthropological and sociological accounts, Japan is a high-trust society . . . so there is something very paradoxical about these empirical findings" (2000: 124–125). Katzenstein solves this paradox on methodological grounds: "Interviews and experiments are often context-free, inquire into hypothetical situations, pose questions about confidence in government (which is low) rather than confidence in state-society relations (which is high), and are conducted in artificial settings" (2000, 125). Katzenstein quotes Newton, who wrote, "It is difficult to know how to interpret figures from a culture which expresses so little but acts so much on trust" (2000: 125). Finally, Susan Pharr (2000) sees a strong correlation between political dissatisfaction and lack of trust over the period of 1975–1995. In contrast, Donatella della Porta strongly disputes this finding and interpretation (2000: 209). A good many of the sources that were interviewed alluded to an absence of trust and confidence in medical technology among Japanese people.

The issue of trust and distrust cannot be resolved one way or another, but it is clear that these factors have implications for medical innovation and medical technology regulation in Japan. The ways individuals perceive and address problems follow deep-rooted cultural and behavioral patterns; perceptions are not spontaneous expressions of public opinion. Charges of corruption make it to the front page of Japanese newspapers, including conflict-of-interest issues among officials, doctors, and hospitals. Corruption charges are expressed in a language that blames individuals, accuses the government of wrong-doing, and overreacts. Going to court to seek redress for a wrong rather than mobilizing pressures on policymakers (elected or appointed alike) to make substantial changes reflects political culture. At the same time Japan is described as a "gift-giving culture" where giving and receiving gifts—small or large—is part of a cultural pattern.

PAL was a real sea change; it pushed medical device regulation further on top of a drug-oriented regulatory framework and a drug-oriented practice of medicine (Interview #48; Interview #51; Interview #12). PAL also brought about an increase in regulatory complexity and legal uncertainty. For the first time, foreign and domestic device makers were affected by far-reaching and costly institutional and organizational changes alike. As sole advocate of PAL, bureaucratic officialdom at the MHLW insisted that PAL was the law of the land and appropriate as a legal framework for medical devices as much as for drugs. But med-tech business interests, through various channels—JFMDA, AdvaMed, and the ACCJ, including individual device makers—early on argued how and why PAL was not an appropriate legal construction for medical devices.

Institutional Change

Within a broader societal context, Muramatsu and Krauss speak to "state power and the strengthening of the state's capacity for collective action" (1996: 215), while Susan Pharr (2000: 316), combining an institutionalist-statist perspective with a social pluralist approach, refers to Japan's tradition of an "activist state" combined with targeted policies aimed at specific sectors and groups in civil society. In this representation, domestic business and trade associations enjoy a privileged position compared to other groups. This perspective explains the status quo of regulation and the observed privileged access of device makers to the bureaucracy, but it does not explain why Japanese and foreign business interests have not been successful in reforming PAL, although various segments of the industry fought bitterly to amend PAL. They finally succeeded. In November 2013 the Japanese government approved the Pharmaceutical and Medical Devices Law (PMDL), which loosened the grip of PAL over medical devices by including a separate chapter on medical devices (Tan 2013a); this is more fully discussed in Chapter 8.

Administrative Reforms

Like other countries, Japan has not escaped the pressures for administrative reform in the twentieth century, and especially from the early 1990s onward. Administrative reform means, above all, an overhaul of the Japanese bureaucracy and coming to grips with economic pressures (Suleiman, 2003: 155–187). To escape "the ills of vertical administration," which are the intense ministerial turf wars (Suleiman, 2003: 165), the government reorganized and decentralized the central ministries. At the same time "the state could more easily act in the public interest because of its impermeability to outside forces" (Suleiman, 2003: 155). Indeed, when the bureaucracy feels that, for example, the pressures of globalization and fierce competition from abroad justify action, it can act without much resistance from any group.

According to Suleiman, the Hashimoto reforms were designed to downsize the public sector, outsource a few state functions, and separate policy formation from policy implementation. But the new agencies or bodies, created in April 2001, are not good illustrations of genuine implementation (as understood in research on policy implementation). Most bodies and agencies that were recently created are so-called detached bodies and include research and test institutes, hospitals, museums, and national universities (Suleiman, 2003: 166–167). The "proposals to strengthen the Diet's institutional capacity to keep the executive branch accountable" (Suleiman, 2003: 167) did not go far. Said differently, the state and state institutions continue to yield undiminished power and influence in politics and policymaking in Japan, including over medical technology regulation, despite the ongoing transformations in the public sector in Japan since the 1980s. While elites are not reluctant to reform institutions and policies, they are reluctant to cede power in those areas. How true!

Based on this characterization and the rich literature on government and health policy, the Japanese state and the bureaucracy are the only viable candidates to expect policy leadership in relation to medical technology matters to emerge. Indeed, the Ministry of Health is a dominant player in medical technology regulation in Japan. Japanese and foreign observers alike describe the medical technology sector in Japan as "backward," weak, and subject to tight controls by central ministries.

The MHLW is responsible for medical technology regulation, but lately this policy area also has become a developmental tool of the Ministry of Economy, Trade, and Industry (METI, previously MITI until 2001) and, to a lesser degree, the Ministry of Education, Culture, Sports, Science, and Technology (MEXT), which is responsible for university education, clinical research, and science. Despite modest steps taken in 2006 and 2007 (discussed in detail in Chapters 6 and 8), the paradox that consists in the portrayal of a strong and proactive Japanese state in the economy, a proactive civil service, and the reality of medical technology regulation in Japan cannot be resolved. A shift in the political-administrative relationship between the Cabinet and the ministries is a likely explanation for the changes (McCall, Rosenbluth, and Thies, 2010: 95–122). Some sources spoke to a reversal of policy leadership from MHLW to the Cabinet (Interview #62; MTLF 2007),[2] but this interpretation was not confirmed by others (Interview #1;

MTLF, 2007). Whatever the real change was, the working out of details of regulation, the biannual revisions of the reimbursement scheme, and the workings of subcommittees giving advice to decision-makers in *Chuikyo*, the eminently important organization for the public health insurance program, remained unchanged.

Public Attitudes and Trust and Distrust

Survey research conducted in 2006 and 2007 by the Institute of Health Policy (2006a, 2006b, and 2007)[3] in Tokyo found a high level of dissatisfaction of Japanese people with their health-care system. Among the sources of discontent, three stand out by order of severity: (i) the quality of technology in diagnosis and treatment, (ii) the level of health-care costs, and (iii) the issue of equality in the health-care system that is in jeopardy by recent policy decisions that allow for disparity in wealth (Kondo, 2007, 2006). A majority of patients are dissatisfied in ten out of fifteen items, such as the knowledge level of non-cardiac doctors on heart disease, lack of comparative performance data of hospitals, and the slow speed of government approval of medication and technology (medical equipment). There is no uniform pattern across different disease types, but the data do suggest an enormous need for improvement (Kondo, 2007).

> Patient advocacy groups here are struggling to have their voices heard. In the US the American Heart Association, for example, has a $700 million annual budget; but in Japan, a typical patient advocacy group has a budget of around the equivalent of $20,000 to $30,000, and is not well organized to promote effective policy change. (Wood, 2007: 19–20)

Pressure-Group Politics, Strategies, and Tactics: Then and Now

American observers see the current developments as a confirmation of their conviction that little of fundamental importance has changed in medical device regulation in Japan since the mid-1980s, and that the earlier obstacles—regulatory, organizational, behavioral, and cultural—remain intact (Interview #20; Interview #43; Talcott, 1999: 20–21). Watkins (2004a: 1) reports the following:

> In 1993, the US medical technology industry won three important engagements in its battle with the government of Japan. Japan's Ministry of Health and Welfare (MHW) had agreed to exempt US companies from new import requirements concerning Good Import Practices (GIPs). US device manufacturers also had successfully

pushed MHW to adopt a European-style product approvals process, which promised to significantly speed time to market. Perhaps most importantly, the industry had avoided major price cuts in MHW's biannual revision of regulation reimbursement prices for medical devices.

This success did not last. In 1992, and repeatedly in 1993 and 1994, MHLW imposed severe price-cutting measures on medical devices through a decrease of previous reimbursement rates, an increase of co-payments by patients, and other measures. The historic advantages for US companies began to evaporate. From the US side, this strategic battle with the Japanese government has continued ever since. After this experience with an empty promise by the Japanese government, the US-based Health Industry and Manufacturers' Association (HIMA), predecessor of AdvaMed, changed its tactics; it began to cultivate relations with a much broader range and number of key stakeholders and organizational actors. This remains the pattern of lobbying today, according to Michael Watkins. He writes,

> The group agreed the game had changed. Industry was no longer dealing with a narrow technical issue that could be addressed effectively through bilateral trade channels. Because industry's opponents had made foreign device prices a hot-button issue, HIMA and ACCJ needed to fight their battles on the domestic policy front. This necessitated a clearer understanding of how the domestic policy process worked, identification of key decision-makers and opinion leaders, and development of a plan for influencing the 1998 price revision. (Watkins, 2004b: 1)

Relations between the United States and Japan plummeted to a one-time low in general and in the drug and medical technology field in particular (Interview #20; Interview #46). In the mid-1990s, a period of severe tensions between the governments of the two countries and the industry evolved, which lasted until 2006 (Edwin O. Reischauer Center, 2003; Talcott, 2009). MHLW began several initiatives in response to pressures from US interests. The idea of a medical device industry vision that was made public in 2005 and 2006 dates back to 2003 (Takakura, 2003: 17–33). MHLW's willingness to talk in the public arena and introduce minor changes in the regulatory regime is a response to the mass media and a growing awareness among the Japanese public about their health care, in part (Tadashi, 1999), and it is also a response to pressure-group politics.[4]

The Health Bureaucracy

Embedded in a tradition of an "activist state" and an "activist civil service" acting in the public interest, regulatory policy is a privileged domain of the executive branch in any political system; it is largely removed from the democratic process and is subject to only limited accountability (Campbell, 1994). PAL gave the bureaucracy considerable leeway and added enormous complexity, uncertainty, and constraints to what used to be the medical device framework prior to PAL. It is both rigid and formalistic, but it is also vague and unclear concerning medical devices. Unclear and vague laws essentially work into the hands of the bureaucracy (Interview #5). The vaguer the law, the more the balance of power and influence shifts to the government and MHLW (Interview #5). Consultations are a bureaucratic tool to control regulatory processes (Interview #5). When issues are vague and ill-defined, the division head makes the final decisions, but the real dilemma is that different division heads make different decisions (Interview #5). The bureaucrats are not nasty; they are smart, but they do want to keep the power. They do not want to be heavy-handed, but they want you to come to them for consultation (Interview #5).

Although a revolving door of lawyers between the private sector and the public sector is unknown to the Japanese civil service, staff in US-based companies frequently spoke about the "more than cozy" relationships between Japanese groups and MHLW to the disadvantage of non-Japanese interests. In the process, I learned about two variants of "bureaucratic capture" in the Japanese context. The first is the phenomenon of "descending from heaven" (*amakudari*). *Amakudari* means that upon retirement, higher-level civil servants can easily change over to the private sector, where they may end up serving in a variety of functions: as special advisers to company presidents, serving as experts in the many committees of trade associations, receiving commissions, running a physician payment organization, and the like. I met several former senior-level civil servants in their new positions who were quite eager to talk once I was introduced by a trusted source. Without referral by a trusted source, there was no access to officials or staff.

Another mechanism that provides privileged access to the bureaucracy is the assignment of Japanese journalists to a ministry, including MHLW. This privileged access means one of two things: first, in theory, journalists can be independent observers and reporters, but in practice, they are keepers of privileged information that is negotiated behind closed doors in a troika of bureaucratic, business, and political interests. This access is denied to foreign journalists. American observers lamented the fact that these two routine practices help sustain privileged access of domestic groups to the Japanese bureaucracy (Interview #15; Interview #20; Interview #23; Interview #35). Big players also expressed similar opinions, but somehow their complaints about lack of access to the bureaucracy are hardly convincing, given the strength of organized pressure-group politics.

Martin Fackler's piece in the *New York Times* on November 21, 2009 (p. A4–5) highlights the importance of this factor to the study at hand. He reported that then Prime Minister Yukio Hatoyama's government stood up to the nation's "most powerful interest groups, the press clubs, which are century-old, cartel-like arrangements in which reporters from major new media outlets are stationed inside government offices and enjoy close, constant access to officials." Prime Minister Hatoyama intended a "grand cleanup of postwar governance." Can anybody under these circumstances expect the media to serve as monitor of the government and bureaucracy? While there are laws, there are also cultural habits and routine political-administrative practices that may matter when domestic companies prepare the submission of documents and consult with PMDA or with MHLW for compliance and enforcement. The following chapter discusses the legislative intentions of PAL and explores the radical changes made by PAL that the domestic and foreign industry did not applaud.

Notes

1. A US-trained medical doctor, Dr. Huimin Wang was the chair of ACCJ's Medical Devices and Diagnostics Subcommittee in 2007. He is corporate vice-president of Japan and Intercontinental Edwards Lifesciences Limited. He shared similar views with me when I interviewed him on May 15, 2007.
2. This viewpoint emerged in the open discussions at the international conference.
3. The Institute of Health Policy routinely conducts surveys covering the entire range of topics relevant to people's health, expectations, and satisfaction with their health-care system.
4. This perspective as evidence draws on the *Japan Submission Workshops* sponsored by AdvaMed on November 8–9, 2006, the initiation of cooperation through the *East and West Think Tank Meetings* in January 2007, and the *Leadership Dialogue for Stakeholders and Policy Leadership from Japan and the United States* in Karuizawa, April 21–23, 2007.

4

The Pharmaceutical Affairs Law (PAL)

Now that the previous chapter has briefly sketched out the main political, bureaucratic, and social forces in existence prior to PAL in 2005, this chapter turns to PAL and explores why medical device regulation was reorganized and how it institutionalized a number of formal building blocks of medical technology regulation. It is difficult to avoid highly complex technical and legal details when commenting on the PAL as policy and as law. Not only does the PAL touch on the organization of MHLW, which sits at the apex of regulatory processes and the public health insurance program, but PAL also impacts the entire community of device makers, the distribution and supply system in Japan, and the collection process for scientific input used in decision-making. The final section briefly introduces the Pharmaceutical and Medical Device Agency (PMDA) as an example of public-sector reform designed to achieve three objectives: to modernize medical device regulation, to improve the structural conditions for clinical research, and to enhance access to much-needed specialized treatments and care in Japan.

Enacted in 1943, PAL was first extended in 1948 to cover medical devices and cosmetics and underwent further revisions in the 1960s, 1970s, and 1980s. As a framework law, PAL covers pharmaceuticals, quasi-drugs (*iyaku-bugaihin*), cosmetics, and medical devices and *in vitro* diagnostics (IVDs) (including veterinary drugs, veterinary quasi-drugs, and veterinary medical devices). PAL is an extraordinarily complex and, for medical devices, a highly ambiguous piece of legislation due to its primary drug orientation. On July 25, 2002, the Japanese House of Representatives adopted a substantially revised PAL, prepared by the health bureaucracy, which came into force on April 1, 2005.

Unlike the Medical Device Amendments of 1976 (FDA) and three EU directives of the 1990s, including their implementing structural agents, the Japanese regime is young, inexperienced, and still undergoing further transmutations through amendments, revisions of regulatory requirements, and reinterpretations of previous guidelines, to the extent that they exist at all. In the mid-1990s, the HIV-infected blood scandal, which spoke directly to the deficiencies in the regulatory system for blood products and drugs, was a catalyst for major legislative and organizational changes by the central bureaucracy. Three domestic manufacturers of blood products and a high-ranking official of the Ministry of Health ended up in jail (Feldman, 1999: 59–63). It took six more years before the principal legal framework was enacted in 2005. In other words, whatever regulation was applied to medical devices prior to 2005 in Japan, it was part of drug legislation.

Consequently, PAL displayed a top-heavy bias more in favor of drugs and came along with an array of enforcement acts, ministerial ordinances, and administrative guidance. It also ended the practice of mixing business and government interests inside the old Pharmaceutical Safety Bureau within the Ministry of Health. Was this organizational change genuine? In some cases, measures significantly went beyond the status quo, and the Ministry of Health was reorganized; thus the MHW became the MHLW. Yet other practices, like the privileged access of domestic vested interests to the health bureaucracy, were not stopped; many routine measures required insider experience.

The Objectives of PAL

The amended PAL pursued several objectives, some real and consequential, while others were mostly rhetorical and never enforced (Interview #15; Interview #20; Interview #46). The first objective was to secure the quality, efficacy, and safety of drugs, quasi-drugs, cosmetics, and medical devices. The second objective was to encourage research and the development of pharmaceuticals and medical devices in Japan. A third objective was to regulate advertisement, to institutionalize the authority of the supervisory agency (PMDA) to do on-the-spot inspections, and finally to strengthen post-marketing safety measures by mandating the reporting of adverse events with medical devices, drugs, and quasi-drugs. These objectives were all directly related to a final, most important, strategic move: to bring Japanese market practices in line with the practices of the United States and the European Union and to facilitate access to international markets.

A Japanese industry expert describes PAL as a "dramatic" and "significant" piece of legislation further "revolutionizing" medical device regulation (Mitsumori, 2007a and 2007b). It tightened regulatory requirements for safety and biologics products; it laid down rules for investigator-initiated clinical trials; it required the registration of medical devices which necessitated the assistance of a third party, a so-called market authorization holder (MAH); and it launched an array of related legal and organizational changes in pre-market practices by companies and health sites. In addition, PAL toughened legal requirements for marketing and licensing, post-marketing surveillance, and safety, including the drug master files (Hirose, 2006a and 2006b).[1] In sum, PAL brought both continuity and change: change came through PAL and continuity through established and entrenched habits, practices, and customs.

One source close to the Japanese medical device industry described PAL this way: "95% of PAL is relevant to pharmaceuticals and only 5% to medical devices" (Interview #28). A scientist expert asserted that the norm of good clinical practice (GCP) for drugs was simply renamed for medical devices (Interview #51). Whether 95 percent or less, it does not matter; the fact remains that PAL is an inappropriate framework law for a good many medical devices. Indeed, medical devices are sitting uncomfortably under this legal umbrella and are embedded in several layers of rules, ministerial ordinances, notifications, and administrative guidance, with medical device-specific instructions scattered throughout. For diagnostic products, the toolbox is even more complex.[2] In a way, medical device regulation was a by-product of PAL, which was primarily drafted in response to the giant lobby of the pharmaceutical sector.

Regulatory Policy: The Structural Components

To achieve the objective of bringing Japan up to par with medical technology regulation in the European Union and the United States, the bureaucracy presented a translated and slightly altered version of the Summary Technical Document (STED)[3] as a draft to the two chambers of the Diet (Japanese parliament), which voted favorably for it. Originally, STED was developed by the members of the GHTF to promote timely access to international markets. It was designed as an internationally accepted harmonized submission standard (GHTF, 2006a and 2006; Kessler, 2007a and 2007b). Participating countries could, but need not, adopt it for *ex ante* marketing approval and evaluations. Japanese bureaucratic policymakers chose to institutionalize STED as domestic law rather than rely on the equivalency of domestic legislation (Tominaga, 2006: 4–5; Naito, 2006: 5–6). Table 4.1 outlines the building blocks of STED.

61

Table 4.1. The elements of the Summary Technical Document (STED).

- Summary of device information
- Essential principles and evidence of conformity
- Device description
- Labeling
- Risk analysis
- Manufacturing information
- Clinical trial data summary.

Source: Yoshio Mitsumori, "The Latest Regulatory Environment for Medical Devices in Japan. News from Japan." *Medical Product Outsourcing Magazine,* January 2007: 32–40, here 37; for an update and progress report, see Hiroshi Ishikawa. "STED Implementation, a Status Report: Japan." Presentation 3 at the GHTF International Conference in Lübeck, Germany, June 29–30, 2006: 23–28. *Conference Proceedings. The 10th Global Harmonization Task Force (GHTF) Conference Design for Patient Safety in a Global Regulatory Model.*

Japan was the first country to write the STED (*Gaiyo*) into domestic law in 2005, but, as Japan's critics would say, not without putting a Japanese spin on it. This spin meant requesting information, documentation, and clinical data beyond what is required by the international standards and the STED. Japan expert Phil Agress at AdvaMed provided insight into a fundamental cause. He wrote, "Companies conduct clinical trials based on an international standard that provides guidance for how to conduct such tests (ISO14155). Japan uses its own standards based on a pharmaceutical model that is not relevant to medical devices" (Agress, 2006: 4). Colby (2004), a controversial interpreter of the Japanese health-care system, argued that the rationale for PAL and for the creation of PMDA was to slow down the adoption of new technologies under the pretext of increasing patient safety, but in reality it is "keeping them off market and off budget."

In turn, some Japanese observers (Interview #24; Interview #26; Interview #15; Interview #7) conceded the spin without calling it a spin. The spin is necessary during a transition period before the Japanese regulators have streamlined the approval and permit systems. Obviously, a spin is in the eye of the beholder. Asked about the validity of this complaint, one official in MHLW (Interview #37) was slightly irritated by the insinuation that the legislation had put a Japanese spin on the interpretation of international standards. He explained, "Standards are published ministerial notes, including Japanese industry standards. ISO standards are translated into Japanese standards. No unique Japanese features are added; the charge of a 'spin' was true several years ago but this situation no longer exists" (Interview #37).

How is the spin possible? Japan supported and endorsed STED at the international level. An industry insider shed light on a so-called post-GHTF meeting dilemma (Interview #23). Every country is in favor of global harmonization, but each state prefers its own national practices (Interview #23).[4] Japanese interpretations allegedly are not uniform. Officials in MHLW interpret what has been agreed upon in two or three different ways. For some officials the important details are X, Y, Z, and for others the important details are A, B, C. For device companies, the only issue that counts boils down to a simple question: what do companies have to do, precisely (Interview #23)?

In addition to the STED, PAL introduced into the Japanese legal system the Global Medical Device Nomenclature (GMDN), the GHTF classification system, and a change of the GMP rules to ISO 13485. While a historical and political analysis of GHTF and its harmonization efforts is not available, it should be noted that GHTF-based decisions have become key ingredients in the Japanese legal system in response to external pressures and has also led to increasing internationalization of medical technology regulation in Japan. The STED is voluntary under the GHTF, and agreements at the global level leave ample room for local requirements and national reinterpretation, which the United States and the European Union and other countries fully exploit. They promoted and signed the STED, but with the exception of Japan, they have not followed through in domestic law, for a variety of reasons. Chief among them are the huge transaction costs of changing existing law and routines, a preference for keeping nationally established practices and routines, and concerns of diminished central control over the regulatory process. This applies in particular to the FDA.

The GHTF has provided key concepts and definitions of what is a clinical investigation, what are clinical data, what is a clinical evaluation, and what counts as clinical evidence (GHTF, 2007b).[5] Research shows that the United States and the EU accept national and local interpretations. Why should Japan not be entitled to the same privileges the United States and the EU claim for themselves? In theory, nothing is wrong. Yet in practice and based on the interviews, the real problem seems to be that MHLW has operated on a case-by-case basis in negotiations and consultations with a company, while the EU and the FDA have attempted to develop soft but uniform and central guidelines on how to go about preparing submission documents and provide more centralized guidance. According to industry critics, initially MHLW did not provide any detailed guidance (Interview #52; Interview #21; Interview #23; Interview #35). Companies had no predictable and reliable way to know what they needed to do in order to produce a satisfactory outcome in the submission process. The AdvaMed-sponsored *Submission Workshop* in November, 2006, in Tokyo, and the discussions in April 2007, at the MTLF in Karuizawa, were meant to provide general guidance. But apparently, these events and discussions were not sufficient. They were largely interpreted as gestures of goodwill rather than as expressions of a willingness to change.

In 2007 and 2008 when the interviews were conducted it was rumored that device makers would be willing to pay the higher fees in return for speedier approval and market access process. User fees are the main financial source of funding PMDA activities; they have gone up not only as a result of PAL, but also because of efforts to speed up time to market (Mitsumori, 2007b: 38). At that time, medical device user fees did not change much, but recent data indicate that user fees of medical devices have gone up further. In 2012, two government reports announced a change of the financial basis of PMDA in the near future (discussed in Chapter 8).

The issue of user fees is not uncontested. To the social scientist it raises the issue of who controls whom: business interests or the bureaucracy? Other observers have different opinions, depending on where they stand and who they are. The idea that business interests control the bureaucracy largely stems from Western scholarship, but scholarship on the Japanese bureaucracy argues that the bureaucracy is in control and responsible for regulatory matters. This may be true at an aggregated level, but reality looks different. When the med-tech industry and individual companies generously sponsored training, workshops, and international conferences in 2006 and 2007, they did not spend good money on charity and altruism. They did so in the hope of speedy access to the market in return for generous sponsorship. What the ultimate balance is between the influence and the power of the bureaucracy vis-à-vis the med-tech industry should be a topic on a future research agenda.

The building blocks of PAL must be clarified in order to appreciate these explanations. PAL stipulated that a device company in Japan must prepare documentation consisting of three parts: (i) the main body of the dossier (*Shonin*), (ii) the STED (*Gaiyo*), and (iii) attachments. If there is a change in the first document, the *Shonin*, a company starts from zero and resubmits (Interview #5). The same applies when the STED or the attachments are inappropriate. In July 2004, PMDA started clinical trial/pre-application consultation for medical devices, but PMDA complained that manufacturers did not make use of this opportunity (Interview #5). Once the clinical trial/pre-application consultation system is launched, the submission process starts with a complete dossier, including a protocol and a consultation category irrespective of whether a clinical trial is eventually required (MHLW/CTIRC, 2007: 17–28). Without protocol, there is no consultation advice, nor are there consultation decisions. A slight alteration of a device, if it is made, must be fully documented again in one of the three categories, and all documents must be resubmitted (Matsumura, 2006). This inflexibility and rigid bureaucratic practice faced a good deal of criticism, and it explains in part why medical technologies reach Japanese patients years later than patients in Western countries.

A root cause of this inflexibility seems to stem from an arguably more rigid and comprehensive definition of when and why clinical trials and clinical studies are required as a precondition for market approval. Interpreting the new PAL, Alan Wilkinson (2007: 109), explained,

> Clinical trials are required to demonstrate efficacy for all new medical devices where there are no equivalent products to which improvements or modifications are made, which could potentially improve the efficacy or expand the scope of the product. Under enforcement regulation 274 of the PAL, clinical trials are required for the following:
> * Devices with a new structure and operating principle,
> * Devices with a new mode of use,
> * Devices with a new purpose, effect or way of manipulation,
> * Products using biological material,
> * Products using generation recombination techniques.

Medical devices are not easily defined and classified. In reality, the boundaries, the structures, and the operating principles underlying devices are fluid. Interpretations range from static and rigid to flexible, and there is an evolving understanding of when the original function of a device changes to become a new product. Does an incrementally changed device generate a new mode of use? An answer depends on the academic discipline and how Japanese law is interpreted. It also depends on when scientific experts and others deliberate about the safety, efficacy/effectiveness, and harm of high-risk devices; that is, in the pre-nano or the post-nano era (Bärbel Dorbeck-Jung, Diana M. Bowman and Geert van Calsten, 2011).

Compliance and Enforcement

To comply with PAL, a manufacturer must have (i) a license of a marketing authorization holder (MAH) and the device company, (ii) marketing approval and pharmacy establishment permits, and (iii) the pharmaceutical and medical devices selling business permits. In addition, PAL regulates advertisement and it institutionalizes on-the-spot inspection by PMDA, the regulatory agency (PMDA, 2007). And PAL outlines the requirements for reporting of adverse events with medical devices, quasi-drugs, and drugs. To qualify as an MAH, a device firm must appoint three distinct controllers in the company: (i) a general manager who oversees good quality practices (GQP) and good vigilance practices (GVP)—in brief, overall production; (ii) a quality assurance controller responsible for GQP (that is, for appropriate shipping and receiving methods); and (iii) a post-marketing safety controller responsible for GVP, post-market surveillance, and the reporting of adverse events.

Licenses

Companies were asked to completely restructure their internal operations, at a tremendous cost. Smaller, foreign companies without prior presence in Japan or those who cannot afford to set up a MAH internally must find a Japanese MAH to represent them. There are few Japanese MAH companies, and they charge large sums of money for their services. In addition, PAL differentiated between four different approval licenses for various product types: (i) designated medical devices (e.g., a cell- or tissue-derived medical device); (ii) sterile medical devices; (iii) devices other than (i) or (ii); and (iv) packaging, labeling, and storage (verified by quality management system inspection (QMS) of the medical device manufacturer). These *ex ante* and *ex post* controls form the essential legal requirements of medical device regulation and for doing business in Japan. Hiroshi Ishikawa, special adviser to the president of Toshiba Medical Corporations and a frequent interpreter of Japanese legislation and practices in international venues, summarized the current duties for good vigilance practices (GVP) to be compliant with the *ex post* controls for market surveillance, recalls, and the handling of adverse events (Ishikawa, 2009b, slide 36). Table 4.2 lays out legal requirements and the primary responsibility holders.

Table 4.2. Legal requirements and responsibilities.

Legal requirements	Primary responsibility holder
Good Clinical Practice (GCP)	Scientists, clinicians, physicians
Adverse Event Reporting (AER)	Manufacturers, health-care providers, hospital management
Good Vigilance Practice (GVP)	Manufacturers, health-care providers
Good Post-Marketing Study Project (GPSP)	Manufacturers
Good Quality Practice (GQP)	Manufacturers
Good Laboratory Practice (GLP)*	Laboratory scientists, pharmacists, technicians, health-care technicians

Source: Good Laboratory Practices: Guide to Compliance. 4th edition, 2010. This definition follows the US 21CFR58 and the OECD Principles of Good Laboratory Practice. Barnett Education Services, Waltham, MA. www.healthtec.com (received 10/6/2010).

*Good Laboratory Practice is "a quality system concerned with the organizational process and the conditions under which non-clinical health and environmental safety studies are placed, performed, monitored, archived and reported."

A team of the US International Trade Commission, which put together the 2007 report, vividly depicts the world of market authorization holders (MAHs), the numerous distribution layers, and the intermediary agents that act between manufacturers and end users:

> More than 80 percent of foreign or domestic manufacturers' medical sales are filtered through a series of regional agents (who often serve rural areas), specialist dealers (who possess highly technical training, such as for cardiac-related medical devices), intermediary dealers (whose purpose and business dealings are ill-defined), and/ or hospital-linked dealers (who directly service hospitals by monitoring daily inventory records, and matching hospital needs with other dealer offerings). Additionally, foreign manufacturers usually also sell through Japan's import distributors, who are considered the most expensive intermediary dealers by Japanese industry analysts interviewed by Commission staff. (USITC, 2007: 39)

One person interviewed bitterly complained that PAL is silent on who is a manufacturer, but PAL holds manufacturers responsible for the production of medical devices (Interview #7). It also holds the MAH responsible for bringing the product to the marketplace. Under the previous In-Country Caretaker system (ICC), in place until February 2005, a foreign manufacturer could bring its medical devices to the market with a simple, one-page application form (Interview #5). Now the process is lengthy and cumbersome, depending on the risk category of the medical technology, and it involves an inspection by the MHLW/PMDA for Class III and IV devices or by a prefectural office for Class I devices.

For a former MHLW official and later adviser to the president of a US company—an *amakudari*—it is crystal clear that the size, internal structure, and capabilities of a company influence the compliance behavior of the company, Japanese and foreign alike. Large Japanese and US-based companies in Japan have no problem with PAL's requirements—they have the resources, the skills, the expertise, and the manpower—but small companies do not have these resources (Interview #7). Presidents of American companies based in Japan know the situation in Japan very well; they are well connected through the right networks, and they have access to the government and bureaucracy (Interview #7). Large Japanese and most US-based companies have a similar structure; that is, they have a boss, a CEO, and a president (Interview #7). They share the information among themselves, circulating it and diffusing it to other companies. There is a lively *quid pro quo* among them (Interview #7).

Numbers about review and approval times are meant to tell a story, and the Japanese numbers do tell a disquieting one. But numbers are also used for political purposes to justify tactics in a long-term strategy of gaining faster access to the Japanese market. If the Japanese data about approval times were compared to the approval times prevailing in the United States prior to the Food and Drug Modernization Act of 1997 (FDAMA) and again with the current data prior to the renewal of the FDAMA in 2012, the comparison would be more equitable. In this case, the "hidden stories behind the numbers" (Stone, 2002: 163–187) reflect the long-standing tensions in US-Japanese relations over access to the Japanese market going back to the 1980s and the selective use of statistics for tactical purposes by US firms.

Tensions between the US and Japanese governments have a long history. In 1990, the Ministry of Health unilaterally announced a two-tiered price cap on pacemakers (Interview #20). In April 1992, the desk officers in charge of drugs and medical equipment at the US embassy negotiated with the Health Insurance Bureau of the Ministry of Health about the pricing of these items. Relatively quickly, heart valves and joints were put on the back burner (Interview #20; Interview #46), and other products were favored.

Compliance with law involves high costs for manufacturers in all industrial sub-sectors. Two product sectors were affected in particular: orthopedic and cardiovascular medical devices (L. E. K., 2005).[6] There is a real irony. Orthopedic technologies and cardiovascular treatments are the most needed by an aging population in Japan. The cause of the higher costs differs for the two sectors. Orthopedic implants were first reclassified in the process of implementing PAL, and costly post-marketing and tracing requirements were introduced. For cardiovascular companies, the reason for the higher costs is different. The cardiovascular industry is growing by leaps and bounds and is aggressively seeking access to better markets. To achieve this, giant cardiovascular companies have intensively increased their staff in the United States and overseas (Interview #52).

A Double Hurdle: Reimbursement

Once the submission process for a device is completed, consultations and negotiations with the bureaucracy are closed, and a device is finally approved, it still cannot be sold in Japan. Approved devices cannot be sold unless they are assigned for reimbursement by the Health Insurance Bureau within MHLW acting on the recommendations of committee-based processes and politics within *Chuikyo*. In other words, unless a medical device is included in the catalog of reimbursable items, a device maker cannot sell his products even after approval in Japan. What may appear to an American observer as an illustration of another Japanese idiosyncrasy is widely practiced in EU countries, including France, Britain, and to a lesser extent in Germany.

For the regulatory affairs staff in a device-making company, a crucial operational question is: where do we start, and what documents do we prepare? Obviously, a logical thing to do would be to meet fully the three-part requirements of PAL for submission: the *Shonin*, STED, and attachments, which leads to an application for reimbursement. Yet apparently this simple logic is not the experience of regulatory affairs professionals in Japan (Interview #5, Interview #15, Interview #20, and Interview #38). According to them, to compensate for a lack of guidance from MHLW, they communicate with each other, share information about their jobs, and discuss the difficulties they encounter, including how these are resolved.

Classification by Risk Categories

Medical devices—both as products and when used in surgical procedures—pose different risks to humans depending on the class of a medical device. As a consequence, medical devices are regulated by risk categories, like in the United States and the EU, though the classes are not identical (Kenny, 2010b; Becker, 2010: 6–7).[7] Depending on the risk category, the regulatory requirements increase. In recent years, Japanese policymakers moved in the direction of classifying medical devices into three groups: new medical devices, improved medical devices, and "me-too" devices (devices with a predicate technology already on the market). PAL originally had abolished the "me-too" category in 2005 but reinstated it on April 1, 2009, as a result of foreign pressures (Mitsumori, 2009d: 1–2; Gross and Hirose, 2009).

Since 2005, Japan has classified medical devices by four risk categories, which were not identical with the categories used in the European Union and the United States. By 2013, the approaches were similar to one another across the three markets. The first risk category, Class I, consists of general medical devices that do not require any approval, certificate, or clinical data. The second, Class II, covers 820 medical devices and 370 IVDs; it consists of controlled medical devices that require a comprehensive third-party review body to certify conformity with standards specified by MHLW.[8] Third-party certification is novel in Japan and emulates the core EU practice and experience, where third-party certification is considered a workable approach to reduce unnecessary and cumbersome government regulation. The last categories, Class III and Class IV, combine two risk classes considered to be highly controlled medical devices that need government approval. Government approval comes in two steps: the PMDA evaluates the application for Class III and Class IV products, and the MHLW, which has final authority for decision-making, gives the final approval. PMDA can only make recommendations; it lacks any final decision-making authority. On clinical data requirements there are two norms: (i) standardized specifications that require no clinical data and (ii) non-standardized specifications that require clinical data. Since 2006, modest progress has been made for Class II devices. MHLW issued an ordinance in September 27, 2010, introducing pre-market standards for 120 Class II devices. Starting in 2012, Class II devices would no longer require a comprehensive review and could now be certified by a third-party certification body (Finn, 2010c).[9] In addition, medical devices that are only partial changes to existing devices would no longer need to undergo a full-blown review, as in the past. Instead, they would only require a notification procedure.

Were the Japanese completely out of line? In 2007 and 2008, when the interviews were conducted, US- and EU-based observers would have answered with a clear yes or a qualified "It depends on the type of product and on the risk classification." Between 2010 and 2011 the US Food and Drug Administration and the Institute of Medicine (IOM, 2011a, 2011b) were reviewing the 510(k) pre-market approval process for Class II devices—based on predicates or equivalent products already on the market. While the Japanese were arguably extremely formalistic in comparative perspective, they were not completely out of line. In a similar vein, the ink on the last medical device directive in the European Union (2007/47/EC), which tightened regulation, had hardly dried when the European Commission announced a major "recast" of the medical device regulatory framework, which means that changes are made within the existing directives. By 2012, the "recast" had become a "revision," meaning that novel legal features were proposed that would become directly applicable to the companies and the member states without having to pass by national parliaments for legitimization. Two proposals for a regulation on medical devices and *in vitro* diagnostics were on the table (European Commission, 2012a and 2012b), and close to fifteen hundred amendments on the MDR and over four hundred on the IVDR were under discussion in the European Parliament. The final legislation is expected by the summer of 2014. However, major disagreements among the co-legislators—the European Parliament and the Council—and the regulatory authorities of the twenty-eight member states need to be resolved first.

To return to the discussion on risk classes and standards, it is unclear whether American industry experts who lobbied for a more efficient and predictable approval and review process got all that they wanted. In November 2010, MHLW announced that it was about to issue certification standards in 2011 for certain Class II medical devices. MHLW sets the standards, and PMDA implements and monitors them (Finn, 2010c). Approval and certification standards were available in 2009, including new review guidelines (PMDA, 2009: 78). In addition, the PMDA issued a notification (1008 No.1) that states that under "unavoidable" and "reasonable" circumstances, "a single representative for the foreign manufacturer who agrees to assume responsibility may submit a single signed and written statement" ("Japan issues minor change," 2010). Previously, PAL mandated a highly unreasonable rule. All company representatives who had anything to do with the manufacturing process had to have a medical certificate (Interview #15). The new ordinance and notification process have streamlined the submission process.

Two interviewees described the health bureaucracy (MHLW) as being in charge of "politics and policy" and the PMDA as in charge of solving "the scientific and technocratic issues" (Interview #37; Interview #53). Japanese officials are perceived to lack any flexibility and to display "zero tolerance for error, the unknown, and uncertainty" (Interview #15). The industry is at loggerheads, according to another industry source (Interview #35).

Moreover, MHLW and PMDA show the same kind of zero tolerance with recalls (Interview #15). If there is a problem with a product, they ask, why not recall it? The company response typically is to acknowledge that a problem exists, but after having the US headquarters check out the alleged problem, the company comes back and tries to convince the officials that the product is perfectly safe (Interview #15). In turn, the MHLW comes back and argues that the firm is taking a chance. The device company responds that the risk that something will go wrong is small. Another industry contact explained that Japanese officials do not make allowance for the possibility that something may go wrong. Instead, they try to make allowances for the possibility that *everything* can go wrong (Interview #35). MHLW has the authority to recall products. If MHLW recalls, it must inform companies of its intention. Medical device companies, like drug companies, prefer to recall a product voluntarily, rather than risk tarnishing their reputation and risk the regulatory authority stepping in. Once the regulatory authority has stepped in, a company has a hard time getting back on track of normal business with MHLW. While robust empirical data on recalls are hard to come by, one source mentioned about two to three hundred recalls of medical devices per year (Interview #37).

Quality systems and auditing are foundational for any regulatory framework on medical devices. PAL introduced the two novel features as new regulatory tools and practices in Japan. Market approval is granted only after PMDA has carried out a QMS audit. Japanese companies recognize that not all is bad about QMS and PMS. But American observers seem upset about an alleged "Japanese spin" on QMS and PMS, and they are upset because PMDA does not have the staff to do the audits (Ludwig, 2006). In 2007, only seven auditors could do audits of foreign companies.

Finally, GCPs are the alpha and omega in every medical device regulatory regime, as it is for the pharmaceutical regime. For this reason, the GHTF has promoted the development of internationally harmonized GCP standards, as previously mentioned (GHTF, 2007: 8). GCPs create an assumption of conformity with scientific standards, but no legal mandate to follow them exists. While the interface of local national standards and harmonized international standards is complex in any regulatory regime and causes an array of problems (to be discussed separately), the most tangible and immediate issue in Japan is the lack of clear-cut legal specification of GCPs for medical devices separate from drugs.

That the GCP for clinical trials of medical devices is almost identical with that for pharmaceuticals or that 95 percent of PAL was relevant to drugs and only 5 percent to medical devices may be exaggerations, but PAL certainly casts a shadow over those who must prepare for or conduct a clinical trial, whether in a company or a health facility. It is unclear what clinical investigators have to do, how they must carry out their responsibility, and what the consequences of the results for the clinical staff and the company are (Interview #28). A few legal provisions are not only ambivalent; they also are not implementable. Informal guidelines for doing clinical trials with medical devices are equally unclear or entirely missing (Interview #28). The absence of guidelines on company-clinical investigator relations (Interview #28) and conflict-of-interest issues stands out (Rodwin, 2011a and 2011b) (more details in Chapter 9).

The same source (Interview #28) explained that when the government wants to get advice, it organizes and stages hearings, but the bureaucracy primarily invites pharma people and not medical device people. Although MHLW recently began to invite representatives of the med-tech industry for discussions, the legacy of the pharmaceutical industry dominating the regulatory discourse and enjoying close and privileged ties to MHLW is felt acutely by device people in the field.

Often, a reference to the term "orphan industry" was made in interviews. The term "orphan industry" can mean several things. First, the sector is ignored, and medical devices are perceived as unimportant in relation to drugs; they do not count. With the exception of the diagnostic imaging sub-sector, the productivity of the Japanese industry in the medical device sector has never been strong historically (Nakayama et al., 2006, 2005a, and 2005b). It has lost further ground over the years (USITC, 2007). The industry sells a multitude of diverse products with different risk and safety levels. Diversity tends to diffuse and fragment rather than consolidate power and influence of economic interests. Each product sector pursues its own interests. For example, the interests of orthopedic and cardiovascular companies are not the same; neither are the interests of manufacturers of pacemakers, wound dressings, or equipment.

Second, in the past, government policies did not promote this sector, nor did they offer financial incentives or give subsidies to stimulate innovation and development. The government only began to pay attention in the post-2000 period. This weakness is in striking contrast to the Japanese car or telecommunications industries, which benefit from public support and the R&D policies in the same way that US manufacturers have benefited. In the United States, public funds complemented R&D funding by industry; most scientific research used to be funded by taxpayers' money, and venture capital has been generously available until the very recent financial crisis (Bok, 1996).

Third, as previously mentioned, the clinical infrastructure in Japan has not kept pace with international medical knowledge and innovations. Finally, the medical device sector has a difficulty speaking with one voice because of the heterogeneity of medical devices. In fact, it speaks with several voices, which dilutes the aggregate influence of the entire sector. There are distinct producer sectors that pray for political attention and satisfactory reimbursement of their products: orthopedics, cardiovascular products, etc.

An anecdote told by an industry source, who wanted to remain completely anonymous, illustrates how PAL creates unnecessary confusion and distortion. The new chair of the committee for GCP-related issues operating within PMDA and MHLW was a medical doctor and highly experienced in pharmacology. A committee consulting with MHLW included pharmacists, device manufacturers, government people, officials of MHLW, etc. A representative of the Japan Federation of Medical Devices Associations (JFMDA) at one of the meetings insisted that medical devices are not like pharmaceuticals. Then the MHLW official, who was in charge and generally viewed as being sympathetic to the medical device community, spoke at length to the risk and safety issues associated with medical technology regulation. The official clarified why and how risk and safety issues for medical technologies differed from those in pharmaceutical regulation, and why the skills and training of doctors were also crucial in the use of medical devices. The chair abruptly said to the division head, "Shut up. If a different GCP exists for drugs and medical devices, this creates confusion." This anecdote made the rounds in the medical device community in Tokyo as an illustration of the dominance of a widespread pharmaceutical mindset in MHLW that device makers are up against. Apparently, the representative of the JFMDA did not step in. "We don't speak up; we keep quiet." He also lashed out at journalists, saying, "Even they don't get it right when they write: the industry side is wrong. How can journalists write such nonsense?" Obviously, the physician-chair was knowledgeable but did not go beyond procedural thinking and the training he received. He could not see an alternative way of thinking; he could not see why the bulk of medical products should not be treated as derivatives of drugs. Over eight hundred types of devices[10] or over five hundred thousand different medical technologies are on the market (Eucomed).

Adverse Event Reporting

A final building block of medical technology regulation mandated by PAL is adverse event reporting (AER) (Ishikawa, 2009a). In theory, AER is the policy instrument designed to secure efficiency, performance, and safety, including meeting the concerns for patient safety; AER marks the end stage of the life cycle of medical technology regulation. AER is a kind of litmus test of whether the regulatory system in place is capable of serving patient safety concerns and whether it can effectively link medical technology regulation and the responsibilities for health-care providers in the field. To enforce GCP and AER, the realities of clinical practice in Japan shape the final outcomes, but PAL failed to explicitly mandate an obligation for hospitals and doctors to report. PAL, a drug-oriented piece of legislation, reinforced the continuity of bureaucratic practices and motivations, but it also brought a radical change.

The objective of this chapter was to present the Pharmaceutical Affairs Law, discuss its legislative intentions, and demonstrate the incompatibility of this heavily drug-oriented piece of legislation with the core features of medical devices. This chapter also showed the embedded nature of regulation in a path-dependent institutional context and highlighted macro-level contextual conditions that negatively impacted the implementation of PAL. From the very beginning in 2005, PAL was exposed to heavy criticism from domestic interest—but above all, foreign interests—and increasingly, pressure to revise PAL mounted over time. By 2012, the time seemed ripe for a change.

Under the DPJ administration, Japan watchers expected a legislative draft in 2013 that would loosen the grip of PAL over the medical device sector and medical devices, based on two government reports published in 2012: *Rebirth of Japan: A Comprehensive Strategy* (National Policy Unit, Cabinet Decision, July 31, 2012) and *The 5-Year Strategy for Promoting Biomedical Innovation*, published on June 6, 2012 (Todai PARI, 2012a). Several workshops based on these reports were held at the Todai Policy Alternatives Research Institute at the University of Tokyo (2012b and 2012c). The next chapter will explore how Japan responded to global pressures, who were the major driving forces, and how international ideas prepared the way for domestic regulation of medical devices in Japan.

Notes

1. Makoto Hirose, in his presentations "Applications for Biological Products" (2006a) and "Notices concerning in-vitro diagnostics" (2006b) highlights the deficiencies prevailing in Japan. Hirose's presentation on IVD requirements provides comparative data on IVD in the United States, EU, and Japan.
2. For IVDs, the regulatory toolbox consists of the "Accreditation Transition Items," "Accreditation Standard Notice," "Notification Transition Item," "Approved Items," "the Handling of QMS Compliance Inspection," and "Deemed Foreign Manufacturer Accreditation," including guidance. This toolbox seems similar to the one described in much literature on the Japanese bureaucracy as a foremost tool of MITI, the forerunner of METI to control the industry and firms in the 1960s, 1970s, and 1980s.
3. The full name is the Summary Technical Document (STED) for demonstrating conformity to the essential principles of safety and performance of medical devices.
4. A comparison of the actions by the FDA or the EU and the EU member states confirms this interpretation.
5. The Global Harmonization Task Force, *Clinical Evidence—Key Definitions and Concepts*, Study Group 5, May 2007 (SG5/N1R8: 2007) was signed by Larry Kessler (FDA), the chair of GHTF.
6. According to a survey commissioned by ACCJ M&MD and carried out by L. E. K., the compliance costs were highest for orthopedic and cardiovascular companies.
7. The Emergo Group reports that the FDA's Center for Devices and Radiological Health (CDRH) division intends to take the review one step further, targeting the Class III *de novo* classification process and clarifying the conditions under which 510(k) applications must submit clinical data.
8. Class II devices—Japanese Industrial Standards (JIS) exist—can be evaluated by a third-party assessment body (based on PAL), such as United Laboratories, Inc., which offers certification services to assist medical device

manufacturer in gaining access to the "Japanese market via ISO 13485:2003, along with local requirements that might apply."

9.   This will affect some 1,788 Class II devices, of which 58 percent are now specified controlled devices. The new rule is expected to go into effect by the end of Japan's fiscal year (i.e., March 31, 2012).

10.   There are over eight hundred combination medical devices on the market, and the variety of combination products is huge. Experts divide them into three groups: (i) a device that combines devices and drugs (e.g., a drug-eluting stent, where the medical device is key, or a prefilled syringe, where the drug is key; (ii) medical devices and *in vitro* diagnostics (e.g., a specimen testing device, where the medical device is the primary agent, or a pregnancy test, where the IVD plays that role); (iii) different medical devices in which several devices are combined in one implant (e.g., an implantation pump).

5

Responses to Global Pressures

In previous chapters, I referred to both external and domestic factors and stimuli inside Japan that were instrumental in shaping PAL. This chapter looks from the outside in, exploring external developments in a global context from the perspective of external actors who want access to the Japanese market. An outside-in view sharpens the observations on the forces that shaped medical technology regulation historically and the main actors and vested interests.

The chapter is organized in four sections and several subsections. Section 1 explores Japan-US government and industry relations over time. Section 2 studies Japan's cooperation in high government-level regulatory reform initiatives with the United States and the EU, then and now. Section 3 focuses on the representation of American interests and their strategically orchestrated lobbying of key Japanese target groups. The final section examines various challenges Japan faces, which are the result of the single European market and increasing internationalization of regulatory affairs on a global scale.

The narrative of Japan's responses to global pressures complements what is written on the domestic scene. This narrative adds further insights into why PAL was revised in 2002 and again in 2005. Despite the excessively lengthy review times and the continuing complex obstacles in the *ex ante* and the *ex post* phase of medical technology regulation, the enactment of PAL and related changes unquestionably have achieved two things: first, they moved the medical device sector in Japan forward to meet the demands by the United States and the European Union for open and fair competition; and second, they ensured that Japan remains a strong and engaged participant in global regulation. To fully grasp the range of external pressures starting with an aggressive lobbying by the US med-tech industry and its presence in Japan requires turning to Japan-US government and industry relations first.

Japan-US Government and Industry Relations

Japan-US relations in the field of medical technology have developed via many agents and mediums at different levels, from global bodies such as the WTO Agreement on Technical Barriers to Trade and the Global Harmonization Task Force, to regional cooperation with the European Union and Asian countries, to direct bilateral trade agreements with the United States. Historically, these bilateral relations have ranged from the well-known, market-oriented sector-selective (MOSS) negotiations between Japan and the United States, starting with a top-level agreement in 1980 between President Reagan and Prime Minister Nakasone to improve access to the Japanese market in four industrial sectors and to direct government contacts via the diplomatic high government-level route. While bilateral activities have been conducted on multiple levels in the past, the central topics in recent years have become more diversified and the contacts intensified in efforts to build bridges across Asian countries and to engage Japan in multi-site clinical trials and bilateral initiatives (MTLF, 2005).

The MTLF-organized international conference took place April 21–23, 2007, at the Manpei Hotel in Karuizawa, Japan. Attendance was by invitation only, but it provided a constructive arena for listening, observing, and interacting with regulators and business participants from Japan and the United States. The conference was hosted by the US-based MTLF and supported in name but not in funding by the US Department of Health and Human Services and MHLW of Japan.[1]

The sponsor list of this event offers a fascinating insight into the kaleidoscope of the medical device political economy, including its networked national and international players in the medical technology industry in Japan. Sponsors were listed by four groups: platinum, gold, silver, and bronze. The "biggies" in medical technology industry worldwide, in terms of political resources, are shown in the platinum row and include 3MHealthCare, Cook, Medtronic, AdvaMed, Boston Scientific, St. Jude Medical, Johnson & Johnson, Siemens, Becton Dickinson, and Biomet. They are followed by the gold sponsors: Zimmer and Stryker, the orthopedic leaders on the world market. The sponsors in the silver category include Edwards Lifesciences and BARD Medical. The entries under the bronze category list either Japanese companies (e.g., Terumo, Sakura, Toshiba Medical Systems Corporation, and Third Wave Japan) or American and European companies that are well established on the Japanese market. While the price of the entry ticket is unknown, the ranking certainly has something to do with the importance of the Japanese market to the individual companies.

Japan Cooperates with the United States and the EU

Japan could not escape the pressures for access to the Japanese market from the United States and the European Union. Prime Minister Koizumi (2001–2006) recognized the inevitability of global market pressures and pushed for a deregulation and regulatory reform agenda in the Japanese economy and distinct industrial sectors, which successor governments have continued to promote with varying success. Starting in 2004, Japan has participated in the Regulatory Reform and Competition Policy Initiative (Regulatory Reform Initiative) with the United States, and progress reports are published twice a year. A similar initiative is the Japan-European Union Regulatory Reform Dialogue in Tokyo, which promotes a deregulation agenda and regulatory reform to reduce the "unnecessary and obstructive regulation" (Ministry of Foreign Affairs; European Commission, 2008a and 2008b; JFMDA, 2006).[2] The items on the EU-Japan agenda include improving the approval process for pharmaceuticals and medical devices and cooperation on regulatory harmonization. As of 2007, Japan had not yet negotiated or signed a Mutual Recognition Agreement (MRA) for medical devices with the European Union,[3] although it had signed an EU-Japan MRA for pharmaceuticals. Instead, Japan entered a Memorandum of Understanding (MOU) for medical devices with Australia and Germany (Takae, 2007).

In March 2010, Eucomed referred to the "device lag" in Japan. After a meeting with the director general of the European and Trade Department of the Japanese Ministry for Economy, Trade, and Industry (METI), Eucomed released a message that reads as follows:

> There seems to be currently a willingness from the Japanese government, including at the Prime Minister's level, to solve regulatory barriers to trade. The Japanese authorities are now proactively engaging with the European Commission and our industry to try to clear such barriers and reach an Economic Integration Agreement. Their objective is certainly linked to the negotiation of the EU-South Korea Free Trade Agreement, which the Japanese fear will have a negative impact on their competitiveness with South Korea vis-à-vis the EU, and probably as well to the current economic crisis and the increasing [economic power] of some emerging markets. (2010)

In October 2009, Japan's Ministry of Health, Labor and Welfare (MHLW) and the Pharmaceutical and Medical Device Agency (PMDA) signed confidentiality agreements with EU Commission's Directorate General Enterprise and Industry and Health Canada for the exchange of information and documents. As reported by Pacific Bridge Medical,

> The exchange of information could include but is not limited to (i) advanced drafts of pending laws, regulations, guidance documents, procedures and other technical documents available to the individual Participants related to medical devices; (ii) post-marketing data and information that could have an impact on public health or information about impending regulatory actions; (iii) information on quality defects or product recalls of products known by MHLW or PMDA to have been manufactured or distributed in the EU and vice versa. (Asia Medical eNewsletter, 2009a)

In November 2010, PMDA signed a "statement of intent" with Swissmedic, the regulatory agency in Switzerland. In late 2010, Japan had in place confidentiality agreements with the UK, Singapore, Canada, the EU, and the United States (Finn and Chalmers, 2010). This is testimony to the increasing relevance of global harmonization and increasing international cooperation.

In a globalizing world, the international exchange of information on the quality and performance of medical products, recalls, and patient safety is highly welcome. However, reserving the information for regulators and the companies concerned while keeping information on product recalls, quality defects in products, and the results of clinical trials (both positive and negative) confidential hardly serves the interests of the Japanese or any public. Neither does it serve the interests of the scientific and surgical communities (Altenstetter, 2011). These agreements definitely reinforce the impression that the most salient information on quality devices, recalls, and the results of trials is privileged information reserved for regulatory authorities through the National Competent Authority Reports (NCARs), the channel of communication among regulatory authorities around the globe. But the international databank is confidential and reserved for regulators.

The activities of the major external stakeholders, discussed in the following section, will show how the US-based medical technology industry in Japan moved from having next to no profile, little presence, and no organized representation in Japan, prior to the 1980s, to building a formidable presence in thriving networks and platforms to promote the interests of American firms today.

The MOSS Med/Pharm Talks

The path-dependent peculiarities—those previously discussed and those to follow in subsequent chapters—along with the enormous price differentials between Japan, the United States, and the EU, seem to have their roots in the MOSS talks starting in 1985. In the talks on Medical Equipment and Pharmaceuticals, abbreviated as the "MOSS Med/Pharm" (US and Japan Negotiating Team, MOSS, 1986a and 1986b), the US and Japanese negotiators reached agreement on a number of key issues that were repeatedly on the agenda in subsequent meetings.[4] First, Japan would simplify and accelerate the regulatory process, and second, it would recognize and accept foreign clinical and other test data as clinical evidence. Third, they agreed on time limits to complete the review and to complete the market approval of new drugs and devices. The maximum time agreed upon was twelve months for new devices, four months for "me-too" devices, eighteen months for new drugs, and six months for IVDs. Fourth, they agreed that Japan would introduce regulations on IVDs. Fifth, the demand for linking approval and pricing mechanisms, so that companies could apply directly to the Ministry of Health for reimbursement of their products, was successful. And sixth, the regulatory process would be kept transparent to facilitate access to the Japanese market. The language, positions, hurdles, complaints, and concessions in the positions of the United States and Japan in the mid-to-late 1980s bears a striking similarity to those included in agreements reached in 2006–2007, except that by the later date, the regulatory processes were streamlined and more closely linked to clinical research and investigation.

The US Industry's Historical Advantage

Several sources privy to the early negotiations felt that the current complaints by US firms totally ignored the historical advantage that US companies gained in the late 1980s (Interview #45, Interview #57, Interview #20, Interview #46, and Interview #13). These sources felt that representatives of US companies totally forget that US firms were allowed access to the Japanese market and to physician-owners of clinics and hospitals, and that they obtained relatively favorable reimbursement of their products then. For example, the reimbursement of a medical device falling under the R-zone reimbursement category (one of several different categories, defined as "reasonable zone or margin") (Nakatoni, 2006) was 20 percent. Companies and physicians profited from R-zone reimbursement. In other words, R-zone reimbursement was advantageous to both physicians and companies (Interview #46). This historical advantage slowly and progressively was lost over time when the Ministry of Health, acting under pressure from the Ministry of Finance, began to cut prices and reimbursement rates as part of its efforts to reduce public spending in health care starting in the early 1990s. The rate of 20 percent in the late 1980s had dropped to 2 percent in 2007. Despite the back and forth of US-Japanese relations, overall the joint MOSS negotiations of the late 1980s and early 1990s had introduced an element of predictability into device reimbursement. Prior to the US-Japan joint negotiations, reimbursement was negotiated between the Ministry of Health and the Japan Medical Association (JMA) behind closed doors, or in the "dark room," as one informant put it (Interview #46).

In a NHK TV show aired on November 9, 2006, in Japan ("Why Is It Expensive?" 2006), stakeholders and policymakers in medical device affairs (including a representative of the PMDA, two medical generalists, and one representative of the JMA) were brought together to discuss the disparity in medical device prices between the United States and Japan in recent years. No participant doubted the existence of the price disparities; however, they disagreed over the cause and consequence of price disparities. A seasoned business insider with extensive experience in medical device trade matters between the United States and Japan asserted that the price differences are due to a lack of competition in Japan. For example, the prices of a PTCA catheter increased from the equivalent of ¥75,000 in the United States to ¥212,000 by the time it was imported to Japan. There are other disparities in medical device prices: pacemakers cost the equivalent of ¥620,000 in the United States but ¥1,270,000 in Japan; and a bolt for broken bones costs the equivalent of ¥42,000 in the United States but costs ¥70,000 in Japan. To get into the high price differentials, according to AdvaMed, one also has to look at Japan's high distribution costs and its three-year approval process. For example, when the United States approves the next generation of a pacemaker, Japan is only finally approving an earlier generation of pacemakers. In the meantime, the price of the earlier model in the United States goes down significantly, but the price for the same but older model remains high in Japan.

Yet a contrasting narrative emerges from a questionnaire distributed to Japanese hospitals using PTCA catheters. It refers to considerable price disparities for the cost of medical devices between the

United States and Japan. Three factors explain the price disparities from a Japanese perspective: first, foreign manufacturers set the price for exports very high (in the opinion of Japanese experts, too high); second, domestic manufacturers and products do not and cannot compete with the dominant position of US device makers on the Japanese health-care market, which Americans have almost monopolized since the 1980s and even earlier, to the immediate post-war period; third, the distribution system is also considered costly—twenty-five hundred distributors (down from seven thousand in the 1980s) seek business and profits. Wholesalers play a crucial role as intermediaries between US device companies and hospitals, not only by warehousing supplies, but also by providing loans to hospitals and serving as "collection agencies and banks," and extending the due date of payment to sixty and up to ninety days or more for profit (Colby, 2004: 98–99; USITC, 2007: 31–45; Fahy and Taguchi, 1995).

How can one explain the lack of domestic competitiveness? It is due to a number of diverse factors: the chronic weakness of the domestic med-tech industry, the stricter and complex provisions of PAL, and high fees for approvals and clinical testing, including post-sales safety measures. Small- and medium-sized domestic manufacturers were suffering from a major handicap illustrated in the quote below, which is telling and on target. Similar complaints were alluded to in conversations and interviews. An expatriate business man in Japan was more direct. He writes,

> The sales team goes to a hospital in Higashi Osaka City, only to run into a huge brick wall of foreign manufacturers with long histories of doing business in Japan. A surgeon says he feels comfortable using things that he has been using for the last thirty years; he also implies that using the same devices is also good for the patients. Small domestic companies will have a hard time, they have less money and no administrative support. Pacemakers are overwhelmingly foreign products. (Colby, 2004: 98–99)

Representation and Lobbying of US Interests

Several US communities in medical device affairs are permanently present in Tokyo. The interest constellation has not changed much since the mid-1980s: US embassy personnel, representatives of American firms, the ACCJ, representatives of US-based and Japanese trade associations, and, since 2006, a RAPS affiliate.[5] Today's audience also includes a few investors, albeit in much smaller numbers than in the United States (USITC, 2007; MTLF, 2007). In the MOSS talks, according to Michael Watkins (2004a and 2004b), the stakeholders within the American government included the Department of Justice, the National Security Council, the National Economic Council, the Commerce Department, the State Department, the US trade representative, the US International Trade Commission, and the US Treasury. The industry movers were the Health Industry Manufacturers Association (HIMA); since 2000 it is the Advanced Medical Technology Association (AdvaMed). The American Chamber of Commerce in Japan (ACCJ) began establishing informal contacts in the early 1980s (2001, 2006). Since 2001 the ACCJ MD&D Office has been a focal point of US interests. On April 1, 2009, it changed its name to the American Medical Devices and Diagnostics Manufacturers' Association. Joining hands with two industrial sectors—medical devices and *in vitro* diagnostics—strengthens their lobbying potential in Japan. The new group continues to strategize and make tactical moves following the pattern initiated by their respective predecessor, but in an increasingly competitive international environment.

As mentioned in Chapter 3, Michael Watkins at the Harvard Business School wrote by far the best narrative about the political dynamics of the MOSS process covering the period from the early 1990s to 2004. Watkins engagingly reports on the extensive efforts, the multiple visits, and immense persistence it took for the American side to get cooperative relations between the two countries' leading players off the ground (2004a). He outlines the MOSS process and names the key players (foreign and domestic, government and business), describes the level of government at which US-Japanese relations unfolded over the years, and provides a brief account of their missions and agenda. The second case (Watkins, 2004b) indicates the Japanese targets for lobbying and the flow and direction of political influence and pressures. Although the cases were written in 2004 about a period twenty years before, their analyses of the political climate of lobbying, networking, and liaising are a very astute description of the scene that I experienced twenty years later. These cases vividly report on the complex layers of interactions and the enormous difficulties in communication among the American and Japanese negotiators. They give an accurate account of the agenda items that were discussed most often, such as the periodic price cuts (first by MHW and later by MHLW), appropriate price levels for individual products, and R-zone pricing, including industry practices. They testify to the differential treatment—perceived and actual—that foreign companies received in comparison to domestic companies. According to Watkins' report (2004b: 2), "HIMA representatives visited Japan [twenty] times over the course of 1996 as a lead up to final negotiations on the revision." Visiting Japan twenty times in one year must have been worth the cost.

HIMA representatives targeted three key communities that held seats in *Chuikyo* (the Central Social Insurance Medical Council): the representation of self-insured private-sector employers (*Kenporen*), the JMA with multiple seats on *Chuikyo* and with vast political capital and influence, and academic advisers serving on *Chuikyo*. Other groups were members of the Japanese Diet and their staffers, leading business groups (*Keidanren* and *Nikkeiren*), and leading journalists in the trade and general press.

The participants from the Japanese government included all the organizational actors who were the most influential Japanese stakeholders then and who continue to be influential today. Specifically, among the participants were officials from the Health Insurance Bureau (HIB), PMDA, and the Economic Affairs Divisions within the Health Policy Bureau (HPB). Both HIB and HPB are within MHLW. The Japan Federation of Medical Device Associations (JFMDA) represents the interests of the Japanese industry, the imaging sector, and the IVD sector through ACCJ's Medical Devices and Diagnostics Subcommittee. Watkins describes the discussions as unfriendly, unsympathetic, and unsupportive of what the Japanese were doing. Distrust and open hostility marked US-Japanese relations then.

An American participant in the early US-Japan talks questions the portrayal that Americans give of the Japanese health bureaucracy today. He insisted that US representatives historically had good access to the Ministry of Health and that the Ministry of Health worked with US negotiators (Interview #20). Unfortunately this relationship has been lost over time, for a host of different reasons. In his view, the US-Japan relationship has always been uneven for two reasons. First, there always has been a tendency of the US industry to beat up on Japan; Japan bashing is familiar. And second, American businesses have a high expectation to have access to the Japanese market and any market, as a right and an entitlement. In his view, over time, the US embassy personnel that were very crucial in the 1980s have become disinterested in medical technologies. They are totally oblivious to regulatory details. Using terms such as "arrogant" and "incompetent," he also conceded that the Japanese themselves are often secretive and nontransparent, and that they use only bits of information against the competitor. He felt that there was really no dialogue and trust between the two sides (Interview #20).

I encountered many representatives of US device makers who did not hide a certain sense of superiority and entitlement to access any market, including the Japanese market. They loudly and energetically defended this right in public, irrespective of whether they had experience doing business in Japan or had just started exporting goods to Japan and other foreign markets. They are described as being ill-equipped to deal with foreign cultures and handle administrative practices, and they have little appreciation that other countries and cultures may have their own rules, norms, and standard practices for reasons of their own (Gross, 2005: 77).

How Lobbying Is Orchestrated and Organized

Today, AdvaMed represents some one thousand American companies, though not all are on the Japanese market. In turn, the ACCJ represents approximately seventy Japan-based American companies. AdvaMed and ACCJ are separate entities. Each conducts its own negotiations with MHLW, like individual device makers. However, there is a considerable overlap in membership between AdvaMed and ACCJ.

Dr. Huimin Wang, who had practiced medicine in the United States and spoke English fluently, was chair of ACCJ's subcommittee on MD&D Group in 2007 and corporate vice-president of Japan and Intercontinental Edwards Lifesciences Limited in 2007. In an interview on May 5, 2007, in Tokyo, he explained that the members of ACCJ use AdvaMed headquarters when they want to get through to US policymakers: "Our bosses are all board members of AdvaMed." Dr. Wang explained that when ACCJ needs to communicate with Japanese officials, it takes "the good cop/bad cop approach in local matters." ACCJ uses two strategies: either ACCJ goes alone or with AdvaMed when necessary. Dr. Wang added, "ACCJ is an extended arm of AdvaMed with historical roots going back to the early 1980s."

Over time, ACCJ and AdvaMed have coordinated their lobbying efforts via the ACCJ MD&D Subcommittee increasingly. In 2009, AdvaMed and ACCJ were joined by the American Medical Devices and Diagnostics Manufacturing Association (AMDD). AMDD represents 62 US med-tech companies, or 42 percent of the medical device and diagnostics companies in Japan (*RAJ Devices*, May–June 2009). In Dr. Wang's view, US companies used to play "strong-arm tactics."

But then September 11 happened, and trade issues were put on the back burner.

However, in 2002, a new reimbursement scheme based on foreign average pricing was implemented.[6] "Saying no" was no longer the right way to go. A more diversified strategy, more dialogue, and more discussion and communication with the Japanese was necessary. Finally, the realization sank in that a PR campaign was necessary and that device companies needed to pay more attention to patients. Dr. Wang's explanation echoes Michael Watkins' analysis (2004b). Watkins wrote,

> The Bain study [presenting the new PR] made a huge impact. The policy-making community and the general public were so unaccustomed to positive coverage of industry that there was a great deal of surprise and interest in this new perspective. The public asked why it did not have better access to interesting new technologies. It began to look deeper at the problems in Japan's health care system. By raising these issues and making constructive suggestions, industry had successfully turned the tables on a number of domestic health care constituencies who had been using the issue of device prices to obfuscate their role in Japan's health care crisis. . . . The buzz surrounding the Bain study's release opened doors to important policy-makers. (Watkins, 2004b: 8)

While the ACCJ speaks for US interests, the JFMDA is the playground for Japanese players and politics. The Japan Federation of Medical Device Associations (JFMDA), created only in 1984 and representing approximately twenty trade associations in Japan, takes up the interests of Japanese device companies. JFMDA is the focal point of negotiations with the MHLW (JFMDA, 2007). Japanese companies compensate for a strong US presence in other ways. Like the ACCJ, they know the territory, nurture their historically and structurally privileged access to the Japanese bureaucracy (MHLW, PMDA, MEXT, and METI), and lastly, they operate in their own culture and are familiar with Japanese behavior and language (Interview #7; Interview #24; Interview #57; Interview #28). The JFMDA is seen as having a representational monopoly vis-à-vis the Japanese government. This has been implied quite often in the field. Yet it is difficult to verify this claim. Other sectoral trade associations apart from JFMDA are active in the Japanese scene, such as the Japan Association for the Advancement of Medical Equipment (JAAME), the Japan Industries Association of Radiological Systems (JIRA), and the Japan Association of Medical Equipment Industries (JAMEI).

Demands for Transparency and Participation

How do American interests view the changes brought about by PAL and other government initiatives today? Mr. Ludwig, chair of US-based AdvaMed in 2006, acknowledged that although these changes were initiated with good intentions, "they have had exactly the opposite effect thus far" (Ludwig, 2006). The issue really is one of PAL on paper and actual implementation. In 2008, the ACCJ requested "greater transparency" in legislative and regulatory work and wanted access and involvement in advisory councils (*shingikai*), study groups (*kento kaigai*), and similar consultative organs for the various ministries and agencies (Clinica, 2008: 14). These demands are truly radical, and if implemented, they would be groundbreaking in comparative perspective.

The Single European Market

While the single European market itself is a response to globalization, the preparations for and the creation of the single European market in 1987 were among the most enduring and effective external challenges that impacted Japan's efforts to modernize its medical device regulatory regime. Modernization and the pressures of globalization were challenges facing Japan and its regulatory authorities as much as other stakeholders in the global medical device community. While a detailed analysis of these challenges and developments is beyond the scope of this work, the reality is that ignoring the implications of the single European market for Japan is misguided for three reasons. First, the anticipation of the single market and the EU legal approach to regulation, which relies on international and European standards as a basis for securing the quality and safety of medical devices and counts on so-called notified bodies for CE-marking and certifying conformity with the so-called essential requirements (i.e., EU law), attracted considerable interest and debate around the globe. Second, the dynamic leadership and lobbying by the US-based Health Industry Manufacturers Association (HIMA) led to increased communication, exchange of ideas, and policy learning among highly networked actors groups starting in 1986 and included experts and scientists from the United States, the EU, Japan, and other countries. Third, the European Union, with a population over five hundred million, is an attractive export market. The importance of EU-Japanese trade since then has increased (European Commission, 2013a, 2013b; Maxwell, 2012).

International Developments and Their Impact on Japan

In summary, global harmonization in the medical device sector is unthinkable without first taking into consideration the international discussions in several forums in which Japan was an active and productive participant, and how they in turn impacted PAL. The first was the Global Medical Device Conference serving as the platform for the industry since 1990. A second and most important body was the Global Harmonization Task Force (GHTF), a joint forum of regulatory authorities and the med-tech industry from the five founding member countries (the EU, United States, Japan, Australia, and Japan). Third, observers from the World Health Organization, the International Standards Organization (ISO), the International Electrical Commission (IEC), and the European standardization bodies (CEN and CEN-ELEC) and representatives from developing regions regularly attended meetings, mostly as observers. Finally, starting in 1994, the meetings of ISO/TC210 Quality Management of Medical Devices brought together experts in the medical device field who worked on common standards for medical devices (Tsukamoto, 1999a and 1999b).

Another reason why international developments cannot be ignored in a study on Japan is that Japanese government officials and industry experts were somewhat thrown into a fast-moving international current. They made the acquaintance of the international community and the regulatory authorities and medical device experts from the North American and European regions, in addition to the Pacific/Asian region. Japanese experts and officials collaborated with the international community actively and productively.

A third reason for not ignoring specifically the EU influences on Japan is that the EU's legal approach to medical device regulation inspired much reform work in Japan and elsewhere, and it explains why the bureaucracy took the initiative to draft the revision of PAL. The EU approach was not a blueprint that was imitated literally in all its dimensions, but it is considered nevertheless a crucial driving force of the reforms in Japan. Elements of the EU model, including consumer safety and liability laws, have been copied not only in Japan but also in Australia, China, South Korea, and South America, as well as in Central Europe and Eastern Europe (Nottage 2004, 2005; Hodges, 2005). Under these circumstances it is difficult to conclude—based on a discussion among legal scholars of global regulatory affairs—that global regulatory harmonization in the medical device sector has been Americanized

(Lévi-Faur, 2005; Kelemen, 2007, 2011). Despite this, imitating and borrowing a few legal provisions from EU law does not demonstrate that American interests do not exert strong political influence in the entire regulatory process.

After the study of various external influences that brought pressure on the Japanese government and bureaucracy to bring about institutional change, I now turn to Chapter 6, which explores how the two agent organizations—the Ministry of Health, Labor and Welfare (MHLW) and the Pharmaceutical and Medical Devices Agency (PMDA)—were organized, what they did after PAL was enacted, and what they achieved. The next chapter underscores the nature and extent to which MHLW and PMDA are institutionally and culturally embedded organizations that are in search of new capabilities and resources and engage in organizational and policy learning processes.

Notes

1.   In 1996, US Senator David Durenberger from Minnesota, which also happens to host many device-making companies, had made it his mission to bring together the "medical technology community—including physicians and bioengineers from clinical research institutions and academic health centers, medical device manufacturers, and patient and research advocacy groups" and more recently "health plans and patient organizations." The creation of the Medical Technology Forum was the initiative of Mike Mansfield from Wisconsin, US senator and majority leader and later ambassador to Japan from 1977 to 1988.

2.   The EU wish list can be consulted at http://jpn.ce.ceu.int/data/current/regulatoryreform2005-e.pdf and http://ec.europa.eucomm/external_relations/Japan/intro/regulatory_reform.htm.

3.   Eucomed (the European trade association of the medical technology industry) reports on the slow progress with Japan in "Eucomed, CEC Meeting—Mutual Recognition Agreements, 15 January 1996." This was a loose-leaf paper collection put together by the staff of the European trade association of the medical device industry and distributed to members (national trade associations and large-scale individual companies), in Brussels, prior to the electronic age.

4.   In a farewell speech entitled "US Medical Device Industry in Japan—Its Past, Present, and Future" at the ACCJ MD&D Subcommittee at the US Embassy on December 11, 2007, Mr. Saburo Kimura, a retired senior adviser to the president of Johnson & Johnson from 1998 to 2007, gave a broad overview of the many steps of a long struggle.

5.   RAPS is a regulatory professional society primarily based in the United States and the EU. It opened an office in Japan in 2006.

6.   Foreign average pricing, also called the Foreign Reference Price system, means that reimbursement cannot exceed 150 percent of average prices in the United States, the UK, France, and Germany.

6

Organizational Reform and Government Responsibilities

This chapter will focus on the Ministry of Health, Labor, and Welfare (MHLW), the Pharmaceuticals and Medical Device Agency (PMDA), and the organization of regulatory responsibilities between them. The chapter examines the policy instruments at the disposal of MHLW and PMDA. To understand how they discharge their responsibilities and apply these tools, the chapter primarily draws on field data and the personal views and experiences of the regulators and other informants. For understanding the role of the Ministry of Health, it is useful to distinguish between two responsibilities: its control over medical technology regulation and its control over reimbursement and prices. The second part will look more closely at bureaucratic processes and operations, the distribution system for medical technologies in Japan, and the various advisory committees that recommend strategic and tactical decisions for ultimate decision-making by MHLW.

The Ministry of Health, Labor, and Welfare (MHLW)

MHLW was labeled a "low-status ministry" compared to the "moderate" and "high-status" ministries, respectively Transportation, Justice, and Education and Foreign Affairs, Finance, and International Trade (Richardson, 1997: 111). What matters for this study is the fact that MHLW has been the apex of Japan's regulatory system for medical devices since MHW became MHLW in January 2001. This move in 2001 was part of a broad restructuring of Japan's ministries through a reduction of the number of administrations and harmonizing their functions. A well-entrenched bureaucracy in the state apparatus, MHLW has extensive jurisdiction covering supervisory, monitoring, compliance, and enforcement powers over drugs, quasi-drugs, cosmetics, medical devices, IVDs, and food regulation. Rather than following the *new public management* as other countries did, Japan was a "reluctant reformer" along with France, with both states using their own styles and approaches to administrative reform, according to Suleiman (2003: 155–168). Suleiman characterizes the Japanese bureaucracy as a "centralized, unitary, and well trained bureaucratic machine ready to implement governmental decisions" (Suleiman, 2003: 31).

How does the MHLW and regulatory policymaking on medical devices fit this pattern? While Marc A. Rodwin (2011b: 161–203), Campbell and Ikegami (1998), and Ikegami and Campbell (2008) shed light on the relationship of MHLW and the Japan Medical Association over time, John Creighton Campbell (1994: 113–137), a most renowned observer of the Japanese bureaucracy, highlights the key descriptive features of policymaking, which may partially answer the questions above.

> In Japanese iron triangles, the political role is typically taken not by a legislative committee (which would include all parties) but by the specialized committees of the LDP's Policy Affairs Research Council, made up of majority party Diet members only. These committees can be seen as having a veto power over ministry policy decisions—or, more often, decisions can be seen as the product of joint consultations among the bureaucrats, politicians, and interest group representatives, who are most directly concerned. LDP Diet members who have specialized in a given policy area are called "families" or "tribes" (*zoku*), and they can bring intense pressure to bear on bureaucratic agencies to ensure that their constituencies' interests are fully reflected in governmental decisions. (Campbell, 1994: 125–126)

I assumed that the politicians who attended *A Leadership Dialogue for Stakeholders and Policy Leaders from Japan and the United States* in Karuizawa, April 21–23, 2007, represented such a "tribe" in the field of medical devices. I made efforts to contact them and verify their role, as they could have provided insights into the Japanese "iron triangle" from their perspective. But it was near election time, and the LDP Diet members were in the process of campaigning. I was unable to connect with them. However, Campbell's scholarship provides good information:

> Specialists in some ministries, such as physicians in the Ministry of Health and Welfare, are formally regarded as equal in status to generalist higher civil servants, but they can rise only to a few designated bureau-chief slots. Most often, professionals are relegated to the

> category of middle-ranked civil servants, who can aspire no higher than a minor section-chief post before retirement. . . . (1994: 119)
>
> By contrast, the generalist official on the elite track will serve in several bureaus during his career so that if he becomes vice-minister or chief of the ministerial secretariat he will have hands-on experience across the range of ministerial functions. Inevitably, though, some specialization emerges—no Welfare official can master the intricacies of public pensions, health-care delivery, administration of the pharmaceutical industry, and public assistance all at once. (1994: 119)

This understanding and mastery are sufficient for preparing and carrying out the legislative mandates, but are insufficient for the diversity of medical technologies, new materials, cells, human tissues, and nano-enhanced medical devices, including diagnostics. One source close to MHLW and the industry gave an estimate of the training of background officials: about 50 percent of the officials are trained pharmacists, 10–20 percent are trained doctors, 10–30 percent are classic civil-service generalists (that is, they are trained in law and public administration), while less than 5 percent are engineers (Interview #7). In 2007, of the twenty-seven reviewers on the staff of PMDA, the primary implementing agency, only seven were said to have expertise in biology; some only had an undergraduate degree but mostly training on the job (Interview #29). In terms of salary, medical doctors are paid best (Interview #7), even though they may never move up beyond being a division head (Campbell, 1994: 119). They are followed by lawyers, who usually end up in the top positions in MHLW, though their pay is lower than the salary of medical doctors. Presumably, pharmacists have the most power and influence and engineers rank lowest in the bureaucratic hierarchy (Interview #7).

The majority of health and health-related functions are highly centralized in MHLW. MHLW is responsible for oversight of the entire range of health care, the medical profession, hospitals, and tertiary health facilities, including some aspects (with some important exceptions) relating to clinical research infrastructures, etc. MHLW also has jurisdiction over the enforcement of employment and labor standards, pension, and health insurance. The Pharmaceutical and Food Safety Bureau within MHLW is in charge of policymaking for medical devices, drugs, and cosmetics. Two MHLW offices, the Health Insurance Bureau and the Health Policy Bureau, are involved in overseeing the routine two-year review of the reimbursement scheme and approving the final recommendations for payment policies, fee- and price-setting, and reimbursement of medical devices by *Chuikyo*, the Central Social Insurance Medical Council, with input from four subcommittees. *Chuikyo* is the primary institution with responsibility for the national health protection program. The Health Insurance Bureau is the dominant bureaucratic player (controlling medical expenditures), with the Health Policy Bureau in charge of monitoring medical institutions, hospitals, hospital management, and related matters, playing only second fiddle since the mid-1990s, according to Ikegami and Campbell (2008: 108). The Health Policy Bureau also collects data on medical errors and adverse event reporting. In summary, medical technology regulation and related powers are spread over several organizational units: the Secretariat, the Health Insurance Bureau, the Health Policy Bureau, and the Pharmaceutical Food and Safety Bureau, for various enforcement and compliance issues, with the Health Insurance Bureau serving as the focal point for the national health insurance program, reimbursement, and price-setting.

In light of a manpower shortage, the question arises: were MHLW and PMDA ready for the task of implementing PAL? One interviewee gave a political assessment of the bureaucracy's capability to keep pace with medical-technological innovations (Interview #35). The rate of innovation and new medical devices is getting faster and faster, and MHLW is caught in a bind (Interview #35). The distance between where MHLW is today in terms of regulatory capability and the actual medical-technological innovations (achieved, ongoing, or future) is huge (Interview #35). Over time, the distance between regulatory capability and innovations will get bigger and bigger, but the bureaucratic machinery cannot adjust that fast (Interview #35).

In light of several scandals hampering bureaucratic action, a manpower shortage, and the dissatisfaction of the Japanese with their health-care system, the MHLW was trapped in several ways: politically from the Abe government and successor governments, from the supporters of a national health insurance program, and from the world of innovations. The same source (Interview #35) explained that things are moving a bit faster in the area of combining electronic computer capacity with medical innovation, health information, and health care. The fields of robotics and navigation are moving even faster (Interview #35). Following PAL, the bureaucracy has created layers and layers of rules put on top of the pile of what is basically a pharmaceutical law. However, PAL and actions by MHLW and PMDA are not cast in stone; they are evolving (to be discussed more deeply in Chapter 8).

The "World of Ideas"

Several Japanese sources (Interview #4, Interview #7, Interview #37, Interview #53) characterized the policymaking universe on medical devices as being made up of two distinct poles. They associate "the world of ideas" with MHLW and "the real world" with PMDA. The "world of ideas" consists of two separate arenas. The first is the arena of policy and high- and low-level politics, including political maneuvering, which all occur within the "world of ideas." A second arena within the "world of ideas" is the "world of science" and scientific ideas and issues. MHLW wants to control both, to frame and set policy, and to protect its turf by retaining the power to issue ordinances, make final decisions, and control the consultation, review, and approval processes of medical devices. When scientific-technical issues are perceived to raise political issues, MHLW is the ultimate decision-maker. Although the scientific-technical and the political realms in theory are made up of two different communities, the ultimate decision-making reunites them.

MHLW officials want the industry to consult them, and the companies have numerous consultations with MHLW and with PMDA (Interview #7; Interview #5; Interview #23). Thus, the pipeline to PMDA, the pipeline to MHLW, and the overlapping networks connecting them are well established. According to these sources, PMDA officials are inclined to listen to industry. But because PMDA staff cannot write ordinances, a device company must also consult with MHLW officials. One informant doubted that officials in the "world of ideas" at the policy level have knowledge of complex technical details (Interview #23). By all indicators, these details are impressive, given the variety of medical technologies. He further explained that fewer and fewer staff members are competent to deal with these issues, which in turn creates problems at the examiner level. Because the examiner has no power to make a decision, he or she instead must refer back to MHLW not just once but several times (Interview #23).

While in a comparative perspective, bureaucracies have a good many features in common, country-specific features are a function of domestic politics and policy, government structure, and the country's specific political economy. The features unique to Japan result directly from the particular government-industry relations evolving over decades in the Japanese political economy. One government official who had international experience (Interview #4) gave a portrayal of the US FDA, the

EU, and Japan, each embedded in the respective political culture and economy. He visualized the FDA as sitting in the driver's seat of a horse cart, allowing the industry (perceived as horses) to go fast. He perceived the FDA as a dynamic player in the US political economy and the EU as leaving the decisions to the experts, according to the dictum, "You regulate yourself, but if you make a mistake, we will punish you" (Interview #4); whereas in Japan, officials want to control the industry because of a widely shared view that the industry will do something wrong.

One industry insider explained what is upsetting the medical device community in particular. The MHLW pretends to follow the FDA, but in reality it fails to act like the FDA. Unlike the FDA, it does not provide central guidance of what to do (Interview #28). He pointed out that FDA guidelines typically reflect a consensus on scientific and innovative issues shared by the scientists and FDA officials. By contrast, MHLW has very limited scientific expertise, know-how, and resources (Interview #28). If MHLW wanted to act like the FDA, it would have to assume a tough leadership role, develop a broader vision of its role, and take on the JMA and practicing physicians squarely and directly. The scholarship on the Japan Medical Association clearly shows that the JMA has opposed any interference in medical matters until very recently. The JMA considers guidelines on medical devices as interference with medical matters.

Ikegami and Campbell (2008) speak to a "complicity" of the MHLW and JMA. The health bureaucracy has steered medical technology development and regulation by a command-and-control mode, without dialogue or discussion. It could have provided leadership and a vision but chose not to. One industry insider explained that the law is the law and has to be enforced regardless of its "inflexibility" and "superficial" applicability to medical technologies (Interview #29).

Review and Approval Times

The complaints of the industry about the excessive review and approval times are not new; they go back to the mid-1980s. No one disputed then that Japan had on average a higher review time than the US FDA had at that time (USITC, 2007), even allowing for the fact that the timing of a comparison with US data may make a difference in an interpretation. Review time in Japan was eighteen months in 2003, over thirty-five months in 2004, and about twenty-two months in 2005. In theory, given that the bureaucratic elite for the most part is recruited from the University of Tokyo (Campbell, 1994) and past practices of recruitment seem to continue, MHLW supposedly has the best possible staff to write the bulk of enforcement tools and discharge its responsibilities for a wide range of measures ranging from registration to market approval and the use of medical devices in clinical practice and treatment. In view of highly centralized decision-making powers synchronized inside one government authority, it makes sense to expect an effective, clear, and straightforward decision-making process. Why are there so many delays?

MHLW officials are defensive and are frustrated about being accused of Japan's traditional protectionism. For the AdvaMed-sponsored *Japan Submission Workshop*, which took place November 8–9, 2006, MHLW officials had prepared comprehensive documentation. Dr. Tomiko Tawaragi, then the director of the Office of Medical Device Evaluation inside the Evaluation and Licensing Division (PFSB/MHLW), explained the reasons for the delays from her perspective: documents submitted by device makers are not properly prepared, in that they do not meet all the Japanese scientific requirements for a particular product. Second, applications are incomplete; they lack a proper description or solid data on clinical evaluation, including data on faulty clinical evaluation. Third, the documents reveal that biological safety issues were not observed. Or, finally, the submitted documents may not fully substantiate the performance of a medical device, or the raw materials used are not appropriate. If any of these items are missing or misrepresented, the application is not in compliance with Japanese provisions (Tawaragi, 2006b).

Japanese officials understand the review process as "a process in which logic to demonstrate efficacy, safety and quality of the products is confirmed based on documented evidences and test data submitted by an applicant," Dr. Tomiko Tawaragi explained (2006b). They understand that if a product is already approved by the FDA, this presupposes that sufficient risk assessment has been carried out and should be incorporated in the initial submission. If the Japanese regulator raises follow-up questions, the device firm should base its response on science and meet the understanding of the review process prevailing in Japan. Obviously, Dr. Tawaragi also diplomatically touched on broader and sensitive issues, namely communication gaps between her office and the FDA and between the FDA and PMDA.

At the same *Submission Workshop*, Dr. Tawaragi (2006a) further explained that Japan was prepared to improve the conditions for market approvals and that her office will embark on a "strategic approach to provide innovative medical devices speedily to patients." This requires several steps. A first priority is to identify the medical and diagnostic products most needed in medical care and which are not yet approved in Japan. Three years later, by December 12, 2008, MHLW issued an English translation by AdvaMed (2008) entitled *Action Program for Speedy Review of Medical Devices*, which became the template for future steps for improving the medical device regulatory framework (Yaginuma, 2009). But what is said and what is done may not be the same thing, as subsequent chapters will show.

Delays also depend on the product type and the stage of the review and application process. Problems may develop from a severe shortage of civil-servant experts not knowledgeable in medicine and pharmacy (but, above all, in biotechnology) or materials, engineering, and information technology. The traditional rotation of civil servants in MHLW does not help matters either, which Campbell describes this way: "Each ministry has an apprenticeship period of five to ten years during which the young official is rotated every year or two among posts with diverse functions, plus a spell of classroom instructions either from the ministry or at a university (sometimes overseas)" (1994: 117–118). Rotation may help in acquiring administrative experience and general knowledge in a system of public administration, but it hardly facilitates effective decision-making in scientific issues or on advanced technologies that require the latest and continuously evolving highly specialized domain knowledge and expertise. In fact, the rotation of officials every two years puts inexperienced officials in new decision-making positions in a division or a specialized bureau. Historically, the rotation of civil servants has been the perfect tool of the "classic" administrative systems to train generalists in Germany and France, which Japan emulated (Heady, 2001: 202–289). In general, hiring specialists in public administration is a twentieth-century phenomenon. In this case, the need for specialists also results from the ever more rapidly evolving medical-technological innovations in the last two decades, and even more dramatically the last five years. In sum, there is a fundamental gap between what is needed and what is currently possible.

Japan expert Yoshio Mitsumori describes the foundational problem underlying medical device regulation: medical devices are often reviewed by reviewers with expertise in pharmaceutical products. There is a "disconnect between the reviewers and the devices" (Mitsumori, 2007b: 36–38). By contrast, several contacts—one close to MHLW (Interview #37), one who worked in one of the insurance payment systems (Interview #16), and a representative of a device company (Interview #46)—saw the rotation system from a different angle. They were mindful of the contaminated blood scandal. In their view, rotation is a preventive measure to avoid corruption and the creation of cozy relations between bureaucratic insiders and industry outsiders. While the conventional wisdom about bureaucratic corruption is convincing, widely invoked by official circles, and also documented in the pertinent literature, it loses some validity in light of two established and ingrained institutionalized arrangements that give private domestic interests a structural advantage and privileged access to the bureaucracy, allowing these mechanisms to work in favor of the bureaucracy as well. The first mechanism is *amakudari* (translated in the literature as individuals "descending from heaven"). Upon retirement, senior civil servants are located in key positions in the industry and serve as liaisons between domestic business and the bureaucracy. The second mechanism is the press clubs. They are only open to Japanese journalists who have a monopoly of deciding which aspect of privileged information from a ministry they want to communicate and to whom. And they tend to favor domestic actors. When ideas and tools are prescribed, they have to be implemented. Implementation is the responsibility of PMDA. How this task is discharged and with what results are discussed below.

The Pharmaceutical and Medical Devices Agency (PMDA)

In April 2004, the Pharmaceuticals and Medical Device Agency (PMDA) was created; five years later PMDA established an international affairs office (*RAJ Devices*, 2009: 56–57). The creation of PMDA as "an incorporated administrative agency with a non-civil service status" was the result of liberal policies and pressures for privatization, deregulation, and smaller government through a reduction of the size of the public sector and civil servant staff. Prime Minister Koizumi (in office from 2001 to 2006) further pushed for streamlining government and cutting public-sector spending beyond the administrative reforms engineered by predecessor governments. As a result of these reforms, MHLW faced a higher workload with fewer people and resources. The number of officers in MHLW decreased, while the number of PMDA officers working on a contractual basis increased. In reality, public-sector reform simply was a shift from the public payroll for civil servants to contracts and a contract-based payroll.

The new PMDA resulted from a consolidation of three previous organizations: the Pharmaceutical and Medical Devices Evaluation

Center (PMDEC), the Organization for Pharmaceutical Safety and Research (OPSR), and the Japan Association for the Advancement of Medical Equipment (JAAME), which in the past had played some part in the medical devices approval process, including the review of product registration applications and clinical trial consultations. The creation of PMDA (organizationally separate from MHLW, but under the same governmental roof) was the end result of a ten-year process going back to the public outcry over the HIV-infected blood scandals in 1995 and 1996. With the creation of PMDA, regulatory and business interests were formally disconnected and the close relationship between domestic manufacturers of blood products and the health bureaucracy ended. This move primarily had little to do with speeding up the market approval and review process of medical devices and modernizing a "backward" Japanese regulatory system in line with international practices. It had everything to do with the post-market surveillance failures over HIV-infected blood products and pharmaceutical monitoring, and it involved US companies exporting to Japan (Feldman, 1999: 59–93).

Ames Gross, president of Pacific Bridge Medical (PBM) reports,

> Many in Japan felt that the organizational structure of the regulatory authority involved was to blame for the scandal, and in 1996 the government began to address this problem. In Japan, new drugs and medical products are not only inspected and controlled, but also promoted by the MHW's Pharmaceutical Affairs Bureau (PAB). This inherent conflict of interest, charging one government office with both regulation and promotion, is considered by many to have caused the delay in introducing heat-treated blood products for hemophiliacs and to have prolonged the use of unheated blood products even after the official approval of heat-treated products. (Gross, May 1997)

The PAB was now replaced by a pharmaceutical safety bureau and the promotion functions shifted to the Health Policy Bureau in MHW (after 2002, to MHLW).

At its core, PAL reorganized regulatory powers within MHLW through a partial delegation of regulatory functions from MHLW and other structures to the PMDA (PMDA, 2006). The principal responsibilities of PMDA are reviewing and approving submissions dossiers for the market, conducting post-marketing reviews, and carrying out quality system audits for medical devices, like for drugs and cosmetics. Despite the new organizational status, the PMDA only has authority to review, analyze, and recommend measures to MHLW; it cannot make any decisions on key issues and central operations that

PMDA staff performs. By 2010, the language of PMDA's mission had mutated toward a "three-pillar system unique to Japan," according to the PMDA chief executive Tatsuya Kondo, explaining the official mission of PMDA. The three pillars are "adverse health effects, reviews, and post-marketing safety measures" (Kondo, 2010: 9–17).

Like bureaucrats in MHLW, reviewers in PMDA initially were rotated, although it never made any sense to rotate staff in a highly specialized field that requires the latest technological-scientific expertise and domain knowledge. The rotation of reviewers was stopped in 2010 and replaced by three specialized teams of reviewers, each assigned to a distinct product sector and family of devices. In theory, reviewers are selected in two ways. PMDA chooses reviewers from among a list of external reviewers submitted by a medical specialty group or scientific society; or alternatively, PMDA can choose its own experts. In practice, the pool of experts to choose from is very limited.

Consultation As a Tool of Control

In *Japanese Democracy: Power, Coordination, and Performance*, Bradley Richardson argued,

> Japanese bureaucrats prefer informal arbitration and negotiations over formal legal procedures. Informality in this case results from a desire to preserve ministerial influence by avoiding delegation of control to laws and courts. Bureaucrats are able to influence the behavior of firms more easily this way than if firms were able to challenge bureaucracies in the courts. (1997: 259)

Like MHLW, PMDA uses consultation as a tool of influence and control. Since 2005, PMDA has improved the number and kind of consultation sessions designed to help facilitate the regulatory process (both review and approval). Prior to February 2007, only two consultation sessions existed. But in February 2007, PMDA introduced an array of new consultation categories, in theory. Consultative sessions are not inexpensive, ranging from $5,000 to $8,000 and possibly even going up to $14,000 when clinical trial issues are involved (Wilkinson, 2007: 94–122). In reality, the practice of consultation varies greatly. For example, just to get the registration process started takes a long time. A regulatory affairs professional close to an American heart valve company spoke to a confusing process: "Our group calls the reviewer at PMDA to ask whether the name of the manufacturer on a leaflet must be included. The answer is yes. We call the quality folks.

The answer is no because this official sees the issue at hand as an inspection component" (Interview #5).

According to three company insiders (Interview #35, Interview #7, Interview #28), pre-approval consultations involve several rounds between PMDA and a company, and even sometimes among different specialists within PMDA and MHLW prior to any meetings with company representatives. Questions are raised about the data. Are the data sufficient or not? If they are not, they ask again for information. Companies reply. This goes back and forth several times until PMDA officials finally agree to approve. Review times are variable and depend on the kind of device. The insiders report that in easy cases the review is short and painless, but with a new medical device using new materials that require clinical trial data, it may take up to three years.

An application for a new medical device was submitted that required clinical trials (Interview #35). It was PMDA's first approval on a global scale, and PMDA was said to be nervous. Several meetings between officials allegedly took place before PMDA ever approached the company for questions and information. As mentioned earlier, the number of meetings can significantly increase, and requests for additional information can go back and forth several times, and reviewers change their interpretations from one meeting to the next. An interpretation depends on many factors (Interview #35). The rotation of staff is one of the problems that MHLW has recognized, in principle, and it has introduced a layered approach to reviews, with plans to assign teams of specialized reviewers in the future (*The Action Program for Speedy Review of Medical Devices*, made available by AdvaMed in 2008). The end result of implementation, in all likelihood, will be a combination of implementing "symbolic" and "substantive" goals (Nakamura, 1990: 67–86).

PMDA started with an enormous backlog of over nine hundred applications, with a staff of only forty competent in medical device issues (Ludwig, 2006). PMDA also suffered from a shortage of reviewers. Those who were on board did not have the right kind of expertise and training. Reviewers were either pharmacists or physicians and had little or no training in biotechnology in the past. PMDA in particular was short of raw materials experts and experts in advanced technologies. The dramatic innovations in bioengineering and information technology in the last five years or so have outpaced the available expertise at PMDA.

If PMDA suffers from a manpower shortage and lack of expertise, where will PMDA get the needed experts in the future? Hiring specialists from the private sector, which PMDA desperately needs, is limited because of serious salary differentials between regulatory affairs specialists in private industry and public pay, and also because of conflict-of-interest rules that ban anyone who joins PMDA from working in the same area in which he or she worked in the five-year period before joining PMDA (*ACCJ Journal,* 2007: 20). An industry source mentioned another major dilemma (Interview #7): even when experts from the private sector have the proper know-how and skills and they are hired, they experience a kind of culture shock. They have no civil service experience and are not used to working in a bureaucracy (Interview #7). Making experts out of civil servant reviewers is tough too. Reviewers should not only go by the rulebook (Interview #35) but should also be able to differentiate more between different families of medical devices; they should communicate more and better and improve the review process (Interview #35).

Two elements for improving the regulatory process are vital: the use of standards and pre-review and pre-approval consultations. According to two sources (Interview #35; Interview #52), in the past, the regulator asked for everything in a document submission but did not give much guidance. Now MHLW and PMDA pay more attention to the process through cooperation and consultation with the industry. They talk to each other and come up with solutions. But they need more process-oriented people who appreciate the importance of the process, not rules-oriented people. Not only device companies need to shape up; the MHLW and PMDA have to shape up too (Interview #35). In a society that constantly suspects the industry of wrongdoing, it is difficult to be objective (Interview #35).

The experience of device companies is not uniform. Some representatives of device companies complained that reviewers changed their interpretation, sometimes in regard to the same product, which can have regrettable implications for the company.[1] Prior to PAL, the situation was even worse. MHLW did not communicate with outside experts at all. Reviewers can interpret the law and ordinances narrowly, rigidly, or pragmatically. But they also can avoid taking any decision at all by waiting until the rotation period ends, thus effectively leaving decision-making to their successor when an inexperienced reviewer with limited expertise takes over. Younger reviewers tend to stick to the letter of the law, and if they are pressured into making a decision, they are fully aware that they lack a thorough understanding of the nature of new innovative technologies. They know that if they make a hasty decision that eventually turns out to have been faulty, they will face serious charges under criminal law, since reviewers are personally held responsible for their decisions under Japanese criminal law—a feature unique to Japan (Chapter 2). According to one industry insider, the shadow of criminal law is over every party involved in the process (Interview #15). If reviewers are not applying the new rules strictly, they are doomed; they face liability claims under criminal law. If they decide and apply existing rules, they are doomed too. They face charges of incompetence and acting like a typical bureaucrat (Interview #15).

While PAL has had negative effects on device makers, not everything is seen in a negative light. The head of the regulatory affairs office of a large Japanese company said,

> There is a chance to prove our case; now we have a chance to show data for the submission, including clinical and non-clinical data and data on safety and efficacy. In the past, we relied on the government for everything. Now we can prove with data that our products are safe. Reviewers have changed their way of thinking about medical devices. The process today is different but is also better. (Interview #34)

Overseas inspections are also targets of repeated criticism. A study on overseas inspections recommended a few changes to bring Japanese practices (mostly in the drug sector, but also applicable to medical devices) in line with international practices: (i) overseas inspections should use the ICH-GCP, an internationally agreed-upon standard, rather than the Japanese drug-oriented GCP; (ii) Japan should share inspection findings with the foreign sponsors and investigator/institution and not only with the Japanese applicant; and (iii) Japan should allow foreign companies more time to prepare for an inspection; and finally, (iv) Japanese officials should communicate with overseas regulatory authorities (Hirayama et al., 2005a and 2005b). After reviewing the major organizations in charge of medical device regulation and reviewing how they discharge their responsibilities, Chapter 7 turns to the role of advisory councils and committees, regulatory science, and reimbursement issues.

Note

1.   The summary of reviewers' roles in this paragraph is based on informal notes I took during the sessions and when talking with attendees over coffee breaks during the two-day conference, unless coded and supported by a source. The final report on the MTLF (2007) also does not fully report on these exchanges.

7

Advisory Committees, Science, and Reimbursement

Advisory committees and giving scientific advice to MHLW are part of the "world of ideas"—a political universe. Their activities have implications for regulatory policymaking and reimbursement. These three topics are substantively distinctive, but they share a common feature. They fall under the responsibilities of MHLW; as the standard bearer of ultimate wisdom, MHLW makes the final decisions on issues that often are conflict-prone, involving MHLW and METI, MHLW and the Finance Ministry, MHLW officials and professionals, as well as Japanese and American regulators.

The chapter is organized into three parts. Part one begins with a description of advisory committees. To know whether the committees active in this field share similar characteristics described by Schwartz (1998) and Campbell (1994), I use information from open-ended interviews to piece together an overall view that examines how they work, who participates, and what the outcomes of their deliberations are. Part two focuses on regulatory science and the actors who frame and decide on regulatory scientific issues. The notion that PAL and law determine scientific issues is not the case. Rather, scientific training, practice, and the technology of a medical device itself are the main determinations. The final part is concerned with the reimbursement and price setting of medical products, drawing on health policy scholarship and on e-newsletters by the industry, as a way to offset the lack of accessible data that are subject to control by officialdom.

Understanding the Role of Advisory Committees (*Shingikai*)

Frank Schwartz describes *shingikai* as working in over two hundred councils, with a particular emphasis on committees and subcommittees for lobbying efforts. He refers to the Central Social Medical Insurance Council and its twenty-two committees reporting to the MHW in 1996. His analysis attracted my attention, since I wanted to know more about the committees operating in spaces relevant to medical devices. About fifteen committees are relevant in this field. They operate on several administrative levels and in different arenas, and they give advice and make recommendations to MHLW, the ultimate decision-maker. MHLW typically rubber-stamps their recommendations (Interview #62). Where do the policy ideas that are discussed by the advisory committees and then legitimized by MHLW come from? Depending on the time period, the answer will differ. An idea may originate with MHLW and end with MHLW. Or it may originate within one of the advisory committees or with the Cabinet and then filter down through the administrative hierarchy. Similar questions may arise in METI and its advisory committees.

Each ministry creates its own advisory committees and regulatory bodies, and each follows its own rules and procedures, creating expectations that appeal to their specific clientele (e.g., MHLW and METI, the Regulatory Reform Council, etc.). Academics often work directly for a central ministry or indirectly through think tanks, which are also in the business of advising the government (Interview #62).[1] Committees attached to *Chuikyo* are of particular significance—the Central Social Insurance Medical Council and its subcommittees: the Medical Service Fee Basic Issue Subcommittee, a Survey Subcommittee, a Drug Price Committee, and an Insured Medical Device Expert Subcommittee, with the latter holding a central position for medical devices. In addition, informants reported on several medical technology-specific committees that are attached to MHLW or PMDA, and on committees working with METI on how to overcome the hurdle created by PAL and how to promote medical device innovation of the Japanese industry.

Chuikyo is the most important council and decision-making body for Japan's national health insurance program and for the reimbursement and price setting of medical devices. *Chuikyo* is assisted by and receives recommendations from the four subcommittees mentioned above, recruited from (and according to some contacts, also pressured by) business or academic experts. At the international conference *A Leadership Dialogue for Stakeholders and Policy Leaders from Japan and the United States*, held in Karuizawa, Japan, on April 21–23, 2007, participants advanced arguments that are difficult to put into categories, but a pattern emerged that resembled the scenario drawn by Ikegami and Campbell (2008: 109).

Two different factions of academic experts are active and influential at the level of the Cabinet and within MHLW. MHLW controls the public health insurance program, including issues specific to medical technology. On one side are the defenders of social health insurance (SHI) and its underlying principles of solidarity and egalitarianism; on the other are the advocates of more competition and market-oriented solutions, who emphasize the need for studies of health outcomes and performance ratings. Both share a belief in universal coverage but differ on the means to sustain it.

The professional members of committees attached to *Chuikyo* are chosen from among individuals recommended by JMA, a professional society, or another professional group. The members representing the public must be approved by both chambers of the Diet (parliament). JMA representatives are usually physicians who own a hospital or clinic. They are perceived as being more interested in protecting their turf than in clinical innovations. In contrast, the clinically and scientifically oriented doctors were depicted as not politically active or reflective (Interview #23; Interview #16). They want to care for their patients; they are not in it for the money.

Most committees and subcommittees deliberate behind closed doors. An engaged and committed staff member from MHLW was proud to report that some meetings were now open to the public (Interview #12). I was curious to experience what public participation really meant. Participation in the meeting was by invitation only. I found out that the public meeting was entirely prearranged and orchestrated following a not-so-subtle hierarchy and sequencing of who was allowed to speak and when. Certainly, to the Japanese participants—MHLW officials, academic advisers, lawyers, and others—this understanding of "public-ness" seemed normal. I was disappointed and decided that "public" was definitely a misnomer.

Regulatory Science

The US National Institutes of Health defines regulatory science as "the development and use of the scientific knowledge, tools, standards, and approaches necessary for the assessment of medical product safety, efficacy, quality, potency and performance, and the role of what is a specialized and interdisciplinary area of biomedical research than can generate new knowledge and tools for assessing experimental therapies, preventive therapies and diagnostics" (as quoted by Yeo, 2010; US FDA, 2011).

Scientific knowledge and advice play an important role in regulation, and there is no universal regulatory science. Regulatory science is the domain of government regulators and industry, and it operates in a highly politicized space unique to each political system. Moreover, scientific knowledge and practice very much depend on the environment and professional culture in which one is trained. Hence advice to regulators reflects such professional culture.

MHLW officials and device companies, professionals, and clinicians from the United States and Japan often disagree over scientific and related issues, forming the basis for politics and conflicts. Since the enactment of PAL, disagreements have intensified. A first area covers clinical data: what does the concept "clinical data" mean? Are foreign clinical data acceptable, and if so, under what conditions? Given the complexity of good clinical practice at the global level, should it be understood as an ISO standard (favored by device makers and emphasizing the engineering side of devices) or an ICH standard (favored by MHLW and scientists and experts with a pharmaceutical background)? The second area refers to Adverse Event Reporting (AER) and related issues. The third deals with the definition of what constitutes a "partial change" of medical devices; what approval or notification pathway should be taken? What specific definition of a raw material applies to high-risk devices? Finally, what measures should Japan take to update the pre-April 2005 *Shonin* (product approvals decided on prior to the enactment of PAL)?

These are fairly universal issues, and they concern the United States and the EU as well. Both the United States and the EU took considerable time before they settled on solutions that were good for the last twenty years, but with the dramatic advances in innovative medical devices, in particular in heart medicine, these solutions are no longer appropriate. The US FDA and the EU are in the process of reforming their respective rules. The assessments of these issues depend on the reference points of each country: the law as a constitutive force, administrative practices, and the current legal status quo of the respective medical device regime, as well as medical and bioengineering practices. Cognitive patterns of knowledge and skills are learned in distinct training institutions and internalized through practice in the prevailing professional culture and political economy. What is a new device? What constitutes valid clinical data on medical devices? What are appropriate raw materials for medical devices, on which American and Japanese scientists and officials can agree? While these questions may appear as highly specialized technical details, they are at the center of conflicts and disagreements, not only between the FDA and Japan, but also between the United States and other countries that have aligned themselves with the EU approach (GHTF, 2006c, 2007a, 2009).

Laypeople often take for granted that scientific laws and norms are universal and that scientific experts use them in a context-free environment. Neither is the case. If, for example, raw materials adversely affect the human body, this means biocompatibility has not been secured. Several elements must be in place in order to obtain it. Experts understand the tests that are necessary to secure biocompatibility (Interview #15). Products manufactured based on this understanding are accepted in other parts of the world, but they are not in Japan (Interview #15). According to this source, the Japanese understanding of raw materials is extensive and ranges anywhere from the definition of shelf life and durability to levels of detail about raw materials and all the way to additives, dyes, and proprietary information generally considered ownership of the vendor (Interview #15). Eager to do business but exhausted from a lengthy and burdensome bureaucratic process, the company finally gave in and reluctantly gave the requested information (Interview #15).

MHLW has been and ultimately remains in control of how these and other scientific and technical issues are framed, debated, and finally settled. What MHLW accepts as recommendations depends on the broader political constellation. MHLW acts within the constraints imposed by a shifting balance of power between the bureaucratic leadership of MHLW, the Cabinet Office, the Ministry of Finance, and ultimately the Japanese government. Ikegami and Campbell (2008: 111–112) explain a three-step process providing the overall context of reimbursement and price setting discussed below. As a rule of thumb, the Cabinet Office decides on the global rate of change in the revision of the fee schedule, the Ministry of Finance demands a decrease of spending, while the JMA and the Health Insurance Bureau within MHLW strongly support an increase. The balance of power is by no means constant. For example, during the Koizumi era (2001–2006), the Cabinet Office had asserted itself as a third influential political actor vis-à-vis MHLW and in reimbursement matters vis-à-vis *Chuikyo*, the Social Health Insurance Council (Interview #62).

Prime Minister Koizumi pushed for deregulation, competition, and privatization of the *Japan Post*, national universities, and national hospitals, "even in sectors where the competition had been considered inappropriate because of public interests . . . [The] decision-making process was changed to accelerate the reform and the empowered cabinet office led the whole reform process" (Tomonori Hasegawa, n.d.). This process was greatly assisted by the Council for Regulatory Reform in existence from 2001 to 2004.[2] This assessment echoes an explanation given by three sources close to the Cabinet Office and the industry (Interview #62, Interview #28, Interview #35): "When the cabinet office is strong, MHLW is on the defensive; and when the cabinet office is weak, MHLW is aggressive" (Interview #62). While the Ministry of Finance prepares the budget, MHLW, upon the advice of *Chuikyo*, decides how much and where to make cuts (Campbell and Ikegami, 1998). Whether reimbursement is low, average, or even better than elsewhere is difficult to determine. It would require a product-by-product comparison of reimbursement cases.[3] Decisions on spending and reimbursement are key factors in health care and treatment.

As previously reported, MHLW and the Japanese government were under considerable pressure from a critical press, a public that wanted more information about available treatments, and the political leadership of Prime Minister Koizumi and his immediate successor Prime Minister Abe (in office in 2007). They wanted to bring advanced technologies to Japan. MHLW also was under pressure from various advisory committees reporting to the Cabinet Office that wanted change. In view of growing demands, MHLW began to understand that it could not continue to do business as usual. By the same token, the Japanese public and patients were upset about the care they received and the treatments withheld from them. (See surveys by the Institute of Health Policy and James M. Kondo.)

On medical technology specifically,' the Cabinet Office imposed central guidelines on MHLW. It took a cluster of political initiatives from above, such as *Innovation 25* and *A Five-Year Strategy for Creation of Innovative Drugs and Medical Devices* (examined in Chapter 8), for MHLW to act and engage in changing old procedures. The cabinet also exerted considerable influence over the debates on health-care reform through the Council for the Promotion of Regulatory Reform Agenda, with its many *Action Plans for the Promotion of Regulatory Reform*. Among the working groups were a medical working group and an education research working group. The members were recruited in part from business, and an overwhelming number were academics in the field of economics and law (Council for Regulatory Reform, 2003).

The call for change and the insistence on a more selective and team-oriented approach by PMDA and MHLW originated in the higher levels of the Cabinet Office (Interview #62). Upon the advice of several committees, the Cabinet Office made its recommendations to MHLW to strengthen the medical device regime, to hire more staff, and to create specialized teams of reviewers to be assigned to different families of medical devices (Interview #62). The source insisted that the initiative came from the Cabinet and that it was not the other way around, in the sense that MHLW took the initiative to speed up and improve the regulatory capacity-building and agreed with the recommendations. Some small reforms have gone forward. Last but not least, the Council on Economic and Fiscal Policy chaired by METI also has had an impact on the public debates about health-care reform. Prime Ministers Koizumi (2001–2006) and Abe (2006–2007) and their successors (Yasuo Fukuda, 2007–2008; Taro Aso, 2008–2009; Yukio Hatoyama, 2009–2010; and Nato Kan, 2010–2011) have shown varying degrees of interest in and energy for reforming the regulatory regime and health care. Under the administration of the DPJ headed by Joshihiko Noda (2011–2012), two important government reports announced the revision of PAL and promised further reform of the life sciences and biomedical innovation for fiscal year 2013. On December 26, 2012, the political leadership in Japan went back to Prime Minister Shinzo Abe (LDP).

Frances McCall Rosenbluth and Michael F. Thies (2010) did a study on the politics and elections in Japan and examined changes in agenda-setting powers by the prime minister, his cabinet, and the ministries from the 1980s to the present. Their interpretation reinforces the interview-based narrative above. Although the authors did not specifically address the reorganization in relation to MHLW, their description of the prime minister's office going from being "understaffed and in direct control of almost no areas of policy" (McCall Rosenbluth, and Thies, 2010: 112) to "revising the Cabinet Law to empower the prime minister both to oversee the line ministries and to take the lead in times of crisis" (McCall Rosenbluth, and Thies, 2010: 113) is convincing and reinforces the validity of the narrative. They wrote, "Several new advisory councils, responsible directly to the prime minister, were created as well. In general, the goal was to take back agenda-setting authority from individual ministries, who had long enjoyed a sort of gatekeeper-role, and to vest it in the prime minister and the cabinet office" (McCall Rosenbluth, and Thies, 2010: 113). However, the control over enforcement and day-to-day operations remains vested in the bureaucracy.

Government Controls: Reimbursement and Price Setting

The previous chapters have focused on the structural conditions, the building blocks of medical technology regulation, and the institutional changes brought about by PAL, including new scientific issues and various initiatives and operations carried out by MHLW and PMDA. This section will focus on device-specific government controls over reimbursement and price setting.

Over the last two decades, national spending on health care has trended downward, including the reduction of reimbursement by several percentage points and the reexamination of the levels of prices for medical devices. This downward spiral of public spending is seen against the background of a stagnant economy in Japan during the 1990s. Reimbursement rates of devices were cut following a certain "automatism" without consideration of a need in clinical practice, incremental improvements of devices, and the stage of the product cycle (Interview #35). Writing in 2006, Gross and Loh (2006: 4) provide specific empirical data:

> Of the 13,311 items listed on the [National Health Insurance] NHI scheme, 76% of the items experienced cuts in reimbursement prices. With regard to medical devices, price cuts of less than 15% were imple-mented immediately, while more substantial cuts will be implemented in three phases over the course of 2006, with the final cut occurring in April 2007.... In the orthopedic market, for example, hip implants experienced an average price cut of 13%, while knee implants were cut by about 7%. Reimbursement on trauma products was reduced by 12%, while spinal products experienced minimal reductions of less than 5%. Other products experienced cuts of up to 20%.

In Japan, reimbursement and price setting are excessively regulated and hyper-complex in contrast to the United States, where, for example, the price of a particular orthopedic implant could range anywhere from $800 to $7,000 (Interview #35) and even higher (Rosenthal, 2013). Price and reimbursement levels in Japan are independent of the level of innovation and improvements (Interview #35) and are seen entirely entrenched in the logic of cost containment (Ludwig, 2006; Agress, 2006). Price differentials are reported to be greatest in foreign-dominated product areas, such as orthopedic devices, pacemakers, MRI machines, heart valves, diagnostic systems, and catheters. American observers see Japan's reimbursement system as a major obstacle to the introduction of new technologies in health care. According to one source (Interview #35), new hip stems brought to market in Japan are reimbursed at the same level whether they have unique benefits or the benefits of a thirty-year-old model, and regardless of whether a manufacturer risked little R&D investment or invested a great deal.

The MHLW remains the "single national access point for coverage and reimbursement of all new medical technology," despite a shift in the balance of influence and power all the way up to the Cabinet Office (Wilkinson, 2007: 113). The situation in the EU and its member states is very different. There is a one-stop gate for the regulation of medical devices at the EU level, while decisions on coverage and reimbursement in the member states are fragmented into several jurisdictions, organizations, and professional layers. The FDA-based regulatory framework reserves all regulatory decisions, while coverage and reimbursement decisions are also widely fragmented.

Health policy scholars typically discuss reimbursement issues from the perspective of costs, total public spending, and health care. In turn, companies must make strategic decisions in deciding on a reimbursement class a device company is willing to accept. The trade-off is faster release on the market in exchange for a lower reimbursement level, or a higher reimbursement level for a genuinely new medical device, which entails lengthy and unwieldy consultation, review, and approval processes. A medical product must be approved and must meet particular criteria for a particular reimbursement class before a manufacturer can apply for reimbursement and coverage.

Ikegami and Campbell (1998) examined reimbursement and prices within a macro-policy and a micro-policy perspective of a single-payer health-care system. Japan's general approach has not changed since the 1990s; neither have the two-year reviews of prices and costs and the related cuts to reimbursement rates, including the upgrading or downgrading of functional categories.[4] Naoki Ikegami further explained at the 2007 MTLF conference,

> The government decides not just the size of the pie, but how the pie is divided, such as the micromanagement of procedure fees and setting of drug prices, etc. There is fee-for-service (FFS) for both inpatient and outpatient care. A new DRG-type DPC payment system has been introduced for selected hospitals, but it bundles only lab tests and drugs. Surgical fees and devices continue to be billed based on fee-for-service. The government sets the conditions for and ensures compliance. The patient cannot leave the hospital before paying the

bill. There is peer review of claims in each prefecture. If the item is judged inappropriate, payment is denied. There are inspections of facilities every 1–10 years. The bill services listed in claims are matched with medical records. If considered inappropriate, the provider must retrospectively pay back the amount inappropriately billed. Regulations have teeth. (8).

These fee schedules and fixed reimbursement levels for all services uniformly apply nationwide to all payers and providers.

As mentioned previously, MHLW decides reimbursement levels and prices on the basis of recommendations by *Chuikyo* and its subcommittees: the Medical Service Fee Basic Issue Subcommittee, a Survey Subcommittee, a Drug Price Committee, and an Insured Medical Device Expert Subcommittee. Price revisions are based on surveys—a national survey of all distributors in Japan (May–September) and on a comparative survey of the United States, the United Kingdom, France, and Germany. Comparative foreign pricing was stopped in 2008 and replaced by a mix of different measures, which took effect in 2010.

The participants in the meetings of *Chuikyo* include eight payers, eight health-care professionals, four representatives of the general public, and two experts.[5] *Chuikyo* retained the power to appoint committee members, but its power was somewhat curtailed and limited to a discussion of the final price of medical services (Interview #62). The composition of *Chuikyo* was changed, and revision of the fee schedule was taken out of its jurisdiction (Interview #62). According to Naoki Ikegami, this move was simply cosmetic; it put something into official language that had been practiced all along.[6] The president of the Japan Hospital Association praised the efforts by the new hospital representatives who were serving on the committee for the first time: "Two Central Social Insurance Medical Council members, nominated by the Japan Conference of Hospital Corporations, really fought well, although they bore the handicap of fighting their first campaign. We appreciate this and thank them for it" (Shuzu Yamamoto, 2007: 1).

Newcomers to closely networked political allies typically are at a disadvantage and have a hard time at first breaking open closed circles of like-minded accomplices. All eyes were on the newcomers when I was in Tokyo in January 2008. They were expected to speak for hospital doctors, including the scientifically oriented doctors. Could they raise their voice as independents, or would they be co-opted into one or the other camp? Ikegami and Campbell's "uneven medical axis of power" may not end after all. Gross and Hirose, writing in January 2007, raised hopes that things might be changing, but hopes were all they had.

> Though some MHLW officials deny the influence of politics in decision making, lobbying efforts may still direct *Chuikyo* members prior to the actual meetings. Also, medical doctors elected by the Japan Medical Association and payers may still have more influence in the *Chuikyo* meetings than the general public representatives . . .
>
> To assuage these concerns, *Chuikyo* plans on becoming a more data-oriented system rather than a politically-oriented system. Features of this new system include a fair system that avoids favoritism to certain medical policies, groups, and products, and conducts appropriate review of relevant data on efficacy, safety, popularity, efficiency, technical improvements, and societal needs. *Chiukyo* plans on increasing the number of public members in the council to bring in more neutral, unbiased opinions. (2007)

The US-based AdvaMed and ACCJ in Tokyo presented the collective view of American companies on how to revise the reimbursement and pricing system in Japan at a *Chuikyo* industry hearing on October 24, 2007. For each type of reimbursement—functional categories, FAP inappropriately low reimbursement prices, C1/C2 products, clinical trial premiums, R-zone—they presented their ideas for reform:

> The reimbursement system for medical technology should be reformed by recognizing the special characteristics of these products as well as Japan's unique market structure and the need to reward innovation. Among the special characteristics of medical devices is the fact that many such products must be made with diverse specifications to conform to patients' various physical structures and specific disease conditions. Also, medical devices can last many years—with an initial upfront cost amortized over its life—and quality is a factor in determining how long. (AdvaMed 2007: 2–4)

AdvaMed and the ACCJ Subcommittee MD&D had commissioned several studies that formed the basis for formulating the most recent strategy and built a case for "leniency" in the course of 2007. ACCJ's Subcommittee on Medical Devices and Diagnostics (Subcommittee MD&D) was renamed on April 1, 2009, as the American Medical Devices and Diagnostics Manufacturers' Association in Japan. As an independent organization, it is supposed to "foster speed and efficiency when addressing the common advocacy interests of companies formerly represented by the ACCJ Medical Devices and Diagnostics

Subcommittee in Japan. Advocacy activities included the preparation of timely policy recommendations related to regulatory issues, national health insurance reimbursement payments, and healthcare system reform in Japan, in order to provide 'global-standard advanced medical technology to Japanese patients'" (Mitsumori, 2009c: 1–3).

Reimbursement and price setting seem to be an art rather than a science. Representatives of drug companies and different medical device product sectors compete with each other for higher reimbursement levels. Each lobbying group seeks out a separate meeting with MHLW to gain advantage. Said one informant (Interview #20), medical device people know their system, the drug people know their system, and the IVD people know their system. But they lack an understanding of the overall picture. Final reimbursement levels and prices are the result of politics, lobbying, and negotiating within the constraints of the Japanese national budget and the government's policy preference to contain spending rather than expanding access to health technologies. Recognizing medical technologies as a component of economic growth in Japan is recent. This topic will be addressed in Chapter 8.

The constant price-cutting of and low reimbursement for medical devices in Japan since the early 1990s have continuously touched a raw nerve in all relevant communities concerned with reimbursement issues. Heavy lobbying efforts were staged in 2003, 2005, and again in 2007. In 2007, the lobbying efforts were successful. MHLW abandoned the method of setting fees on the basis of average foreign prices. It is no longer included in the fee structure that took effect on April 1, 2010. The fee structure now includes enhanced reimbursement for advanced medical technologies. Close observers of the Asian scene suggest that "more medical device categories will be added so the fee structure more closely matches those in other countries" (Ames and Gross, 2009: 1).

Mixed billing (combining insured and non-insured services) was introduced in 2005 with a target set of one hundred procedures and two thousand participating institutions. Implementation was slow. By 2006, only seven procedures were performed in sixty-three institutions, and new technologies were not forthcoming; medical devices need to be approved before they are eligible for mixed billing (Mitsumori, 2006a: 35). Prior to the introduction of mixed billing, a Japanese patient who wanted to pay the difference between what was and what was not covered by the national health insurance program lost coverage completely, leaving the patient to pay the entire bill (MTLF, 2007).

Interviews did not help to resolve the issue of whether reimbursement and price setting in Japan are significantly lower than in other countries. Opinions ranged broadly. For example, old and new pacemakers are reimbursed at the same rate. There is no room for profits (Interview #36). The reimbursement of MRIs in Japan is said to be much lower than in other advanced countries. In fact, it is a sixth of the reimbursement level in the United States and one-third that of Singapore (Interview #28; Interview #25; Interview #20).

Hospital Reimbursement and Fee-for-Service: To Whose Advantage?

Japan moved toward diagnostic procedure combinations (DPCs) to reimburse hospitals in 2003. It extended DPCs to 306 hospitals representing about a quarter of all hospital beds in Japan in 2006. Patient classification is calculated on the basis of diagnosis and procedures, and hospitals receive payments depending on the length of stay at fixed cost. Earlier, reference was made to bundled hospital fees (i.e., the portion assigned to room and board, nursing, and laboratory costs) leaving doctors' fees (for surgery, evaluation, management, and rehabilitation) and outpatient fees to a traditional fee-for-service system. Tatara and Okamoto (2009: 67–68) wrote in an official report on Japan that the implementation of the DPC system nationally was hampered by the limited information system in hospitals on costs and diagnosis. Few hospitals have cost data or accurate records of patient diagnoses (Interview #36). For DPC to function, professional hospital management and analytical capabilities, which are in scarce supply in Japan, are required (Interview #43; Interview #36). Doctors are in charge and are challenged neither by their patients nor by the government or their peers. What little hospital management there is, it is not understood in most cases, and a real vacuum of management knowledge and expertise exists (Interview #36). Yet a vacuum also offers an opportunity for hospitals to collaborate (Interview #36). However, it may take another five to ten years before hospitals will be ready (Wocher, 2007, 2004, and 1999; Wengstrand et al., 2005).

An economic consultant in Tokyo felt that hospital operators have a good understanding of the revenue side, but they fail to understand the cost side, let alone how costs are associated with revenues. Cost data in Japanese hospitals do not exist. Under these circumstances DPC cannot work (Interview #36). This is why the Japanese government introduced the DPC as an experiment first: to prepare the path for the adoption of DRGs in about five to ten years (Interview #36). Physicians thoroughly dislike DPCs (Interview #19), and they continue to receive fee-for service reimbursement differentiated for surgery, high-risk surgery, and other considerations, as previously mentioned.

By way of summary, this chapter discussed advisory committees, issues related to regulatory science, and hospital reimbursement, a most salient aspect of medical technology regulation. Regulation is super-complex, conflict-laden, and intrinsically linked to economic and professional interests. What may be variable in Japan compared to other advanced societies is perhaps the style, the actor constellation, and how science is brought to bear on regulation. Finally, the chapter discussed the central controls over reimbursement and price setting that affect device companies as much as providers of care and treatments. The mechanisms to reimbursement and price setting in numerous committees of *Chuikyo* and MHLW, such as the biannual reimbursement reviews, reexaminations, and repricing, are unique to Japan. Over time, cost and price controls have had priority over improving the quality of care and treatment available to Japanese patients. Japan is by no means alone in its cost-cutting mode. Governments, sickness funds, and private for-profit health insurance companies alike have actively pursued such policies in many countries. The next chapter will focus on the new initiatives to bring new medical devices to Japanese patients.

Notes

1. Chief among the think tanks are Mitsubishi Institute, Fuji General Institute, and UFJ Institute Ltd.
2. The Council for Regulatory Reform, in existence from April 2001 to March 2004, was renamed the Council for Promotion of Regulatory Reform. It was convened again in April 2004 until December 2006.
3. Empirical information is hard to come by. The 2007 study by the USITC and the chapter written by Alan Wilkinson (2007) provides very general data on reimbursement, but not in detail.
4. In 2003 and through 2008, reimbursement rested on six different elements. First, functional categories for groups of devices were used. The initially assigned price was crucial. A second element was foreign average pricing (FAP), which was applied until 2010. A third component covered measures to address products with inappropriately low reimbursement prices. A fourth category included so-called C1/C2 products, which covered the most innovative and advanced medical devices. The fifth category was the most complex and referred to a change of three types of premiums: (a) innovativeness, (b) two different understandings of usefulness and of marketability, and (c) reimbursement category for devices not yet on the Japanese market. A final reimbursement type was class F. This class applied when no equivalent technology or technical fee existed in the Japanese

reimbursement system. The prices and price lists are not disclosed because of their confidential nature.

5. The payers represent the government and payer associations. The health-care professionals include five medical doctors, two dentists (though this privilege has ended as a result of a scandal), and one pharmacist. The general public representatives are academics and professional society members. Of the seven representatives that JMA appoints, five represent practicing physicians and physician-owners of hospitals, and the remaining two are now representatives of hospital associations.

6. Conversation with Professor Naoki Ikegami on January 9, 2008, in Tokyo at the Department of Health Policy and Management, Keio University, Tokyo.

8

Initiatives, Operations, and Processes

To understand the policy, institutional, and organizational changes that have been made and to determine whether they closed the "device lag" and improved regulatory capacities and processes, this chapter focuses on government plans and strategies to address the underdeveloped stage of access to advanced medical therapies. Current and future progress hinges on two poles: medical practice and clinical skills, and innovative and novel medical devices of the domestic industry. The chapter is divided into several parts. The first part begins with a brief discussion to show how a "device lag" in Japan is interdependent with medical practice and a lack of standardized medical procedures in specialty medicine. The second part explores a range of policy and administrative initiatives and activities undertaken jointly by three ministries—MHLW, METI, and MEXT. The aim is to promote innovation creation, close the "device lag" in Japan, and overcome the multiple obstacles to speedy implementation and desired outcomes. A final part clarifies whether the politics or policy initiatives explain ongoing administrative activities.

Improving the "Device Lag" and Access to Advanced Therapies

The concept "device lag" has multiple meanings. A "device lag" (*debaisū-ragū*) most commonly refers to the absence of medical devices and IVDs in Japan that are used in other advanced societies. In Japan, "device lags" are the most acute in oncology, cardiovascular diseases, and orthopedics—the leading diseases (Tatara and Okamoto, 2009: 55). To complicate matters, the concept "device lag" also may refer to an intractable problem in the practice of medicine. The problem is the so-called off-label use of a medical device by a doctor in clinical procedures and treatments. Here two situations need to be differentiated: first, a medical device is not approved in Japan for a particular procedure, which then illustrates an unauthorized use of a device (Eno, 2006). And second, a medical device is used by a doctor in ways "not intended by the manufacturer," which raises legal issues under liability law. The industry is uniquely interested in a "device lag" that stands for the physical absence of a product on the Japanese market, but a "device lag" is or should be of interest to the regulatory authority and the medical profession.

Some evidence from the field, albeit spotty and anecdotal, suggests that the so-called off-label use of medical devices is more of a problem in Japan than in other advanced societies; it may also be more widespread in other countries than commonly assumed, surmised a surgeon (Swiontkowski, 2007; MTLF, 2007: 18). Sources close to companies and the MHLW insist that the incidence of "off-label" uses in clinical practice is indeed higher in Japan than in other advanced industrialized societies (Interview #15, Interview #35, Interview #51). Some feel that the "off-label" use may be encouraged by aggressive salesmanship; others feel device companies could do something about it, but they choose to ignore it. Still others defend device companies, arguing that they have no control over doctors and medical practice.

These explanations may be on target, but alternative explanations are equally plausible. First, an "off-label" use may be a by-product of the policies on medical technology regulation, the politics of MHLW, and its unwillingness to step on the toes of the JMA and physicians. Second, the constraints of cost containment over the last twenty years may contribute to medical creativity and experimentation. Medical experimentation knows no limits. Third, the practice of reimbursing medical devices may have something to do with an elevated "off-label" use. The reimbursement system excludes "devices, surgical operations, and high cost materials from the bundled fee and [are] paid for on a fee-for-service basis at this time" (Shiraishi, 2007: 18–19). This incentive structure benefits physicians and device companies alike. A fourth reason may be the inadequate training of specialty physicians, such as cardiologists (Minami, 2004), health staff, nurses, and technical support staff. Inadequate training may also be a cause of medical errors (explored in Chapter 9). A fifth reason for "off-label" uses may be associated with the business practices of US device makers (Demske, 2008; Feder, 2007; West, 2007). In the United States, they stand accused of giving kickbacks, discounts, and gifts to hospitals and physicians in exchange for brand loyalty of devices and heavy equipment. Why would the industry change its business practices when they do business abroad? The high costs for marketing and doing business in Japan may reflect such business expenses (L. E. K., Analysis, 2005: 22–24).

Several contacts in the field felt that the relationship between physicians and device companies was indeed questionable, but they would not elaborate much further, even when encouraged to do so. The 2007 investigations by the Justice Department of orthopedic and cardiovascular companies in the United States and Marc A. Rodwin's study (2011a: 195) indicate how such incentive structures play into physician-company relations. Physicians have no "*direct* financial incentives to increase revenue or decrease costs," but they have "*indirect* incentives to advance their employer's economic interests" (Rodwin, 2011a: 177). Furthermore, Marc A. Rodwin writes,

> Gifts are important in Japanese culture and business. The boundary between acceptable gifts and illegal kickbacks has shifted over time. So have the kinds of relationships that exist between independent firms. Many supplier-purchaser relationships are termed *Tachiai*— one of mutual dependence. Rather than selling products in individual impersonal transactions, suppliers include extensive support. The purchaser depends on the seller and it is hard to distinguish between the purchased product and service from additional tie-ins. There is no clear line between what is purchased, product support that is provided for free gifts, favors based on a personal or business relationship, and kickbacks. (2011a: 195)

Several anecdotes from field contacts (Interview #43; Interview #57; Interview #40), including a radiologist (Interview #64), are in line with Rodwin's observations (2011a, 2011b). They explained why the number of CTs, MRIs, and PETs per inhabitant is so much higher in Japan than it is in the United States and elsewhere. However, they also pointed out that high-end products (e.g., the diagnostic performance of coronary angiography by 64-row CT and 3 Tesla [3T] MRI scan) are absent in Japan. Since examinations with these technologies are "semi-automatically" covered by the medical insurance program, no one monitors whether such exams are necessary. Managers and owners of small and medium-sized private medical institutions purchase CTs and MRIs and pressure physicians to prescribe diagnostic tests more than medically necessary.

Leaving behind the gray zones of "off-label" use, monetary incentives, medical entrepreneurship, overuse of diagnostic tests, etc., I now turn to the recent initiatives and operations launched by the Japanese government to bring medical technologies and advanced treatments to Japanese patients faster than in the past.

Administrative Reforms and Distinct Instruments

As will be recalled, MHLW and PMDA invariably had come under increasing attack by critiques from the inside and outside of Japan, not only for the long delays of market approvals, but also for the super-complex and cumbersome regulatory process and for providing little reliable guidance or transparent criteria. By 2006, AdvaMed, ACCJ, individual US companies, and Japanese lobbyists were successful in persuading MHLW to participate in an AdvaMed-sponsored *Japanese Submissions Workshop* entitled *How to Comply with Japan's Regulatory Requirements: Strategies for Success,* on November 8–9, 2006, in Tokyo. The agenda covered the entire spectrum of pre-market and post-market responsibilities mandated by PAL, including subsequent and earlier regulations, notifications, etc. A similar initiative was taken by the Japanese Federation of Medical Device Associations on December 11, 2006.

Japanese officials were cautious and firm, but they wanted to be seen as being transparent, open, and fair. Having prepared meticulously written documents and sophisticated PowerPoint presentations, they willingly gave extensive and comprehensive instructions of what to do, how to do it, and when. Admittedly, the PowerPoint presentations discussed technical details in bureaucratic and legalistic language— to be expected from a genuine bureaucracy. That representatives of American business, though fairly subdued and civil at the conference itself, do not seem to care much about business traditions in other countries does not help matters either. Many seem to make little, if any, effort to familiarize themselves with local conditions, the law of the host country, or the language. They come off as arrogant and display a sense of superiority to sell their products in Japan at all costs, as a matter of entitlement. A cultural divide between American business traditions and Japanese culture runs deep, with long roots in the past.

Behind the massive criticism from US lobbyists and device companies are not only irreconcilable cultural and linguistic differences, but also fundamental political differences. Because many technical issues cannot be resolved bureaucratically, they made it to the top of the US-Japan agenda at the highest governmental level. For example, the key thrust of the Abe-Bush accords (April 28, 2007) was to "enhance efforts to promote and protect [intellectual property rights], strengthen energy security, make trade flows more secure and efficient, and increase transparency of governmental regulatory procedures" (Ministry of Foreign Affairs, 2007: 15). Transparency is hardly objectionable, but IPR and standards that define what is "secure and efficient" certainly are.

Acutely aware of the "device lag" and eager to close it by the year 2013, the Japanese government launched a moderately ambitious program on *Innovation 25* and a *Five-Year Strategy for Creation of Innovative Drugs and Medical Devices* [1] (The Prime Minister and His Cabinet, 2007). The two initiatives pursued two distinct objectives: first, stimulating the Japanese economy through the development and presentation of a "medical device industry vision" (Takakura, 2003) and promoting entrepreneurship of Japanese device makers and strengthening R&D; and second, stimulating clinical trials and streamlining the review process for new medical devices. While the former was to be implemented through a medical-engineering initiative under the leadership of METI, the latter was to target clinical research through *"clinical research revitalization"* and the promotion of *"medical institutions and clinical researchers collaborating in clinical trials"* under the leadership of MHLW (MTLF, 2007: 5–6, italics in original). *The Five-Year Strategy,* which was decided by the Health Care Innovation Council on June 6, 2012, was renewed by a Cabinet decision on July 31, 2012, along similar priorities in the health field and the life sciences (National Policy Unit, Cabinet Decision, July 2012; UNDESA, ESCAP, ILO, UNEP, 2012: 39–46).

In a globalizing world, even the staunchest bureaucracy adapts to new circumstances. In 2011, the PMDA published "International Vision," which recognizes the growing interdependence of Japanese regulatory activities with partners abroad and the need for better cooperation with regulatory authorities and foreign researchers. It addresses several focus areas: for example, more efficient communication with the outside world through "accurate English" translations and a higher number of translations, responses to advanced science and technology, and upgrading international operations (e.g., recruiting more staff) (PMDA, 2009 and 2010). The "International Vision" was enhanced with the "PMDA International Vision Roadmap," which places heavy emphasis on concrete steps to achieve the previously stated goals (Yeo, 2013).

MHLW-Based Operations

In early October 2006, MHLW set up a "Study Group on the Early Approval of Medical Devices in Great Need," which consisted of a selection working group (WG) and a study group (SG) for evaluation. They were responsible for putting together a list of highly needed medical devices to be imported in Japan through a fast-track regulatory approval. The groups met for the first time on October 26, 2006. Upon request by the Medical Device Evaluation Office (PFSB/MHLW) and endorsed by the Health Policy Bureau (HPB/MHLW), Japanese scientific and academic societies were asked to submit a prioritized list of highly needed medical devices for early approval. In a step-by-step process, medical devices were ranked and prioritized according to two criteria: "highly medically needed" and "disease severity" (Pharma Japan, 2006). Originally, MHLW intended to approve five or six kinds of medical devices, but by January 2007, after 114 recommendations were received from thirty-eight medical societies, the priority list included thirteen candidates (Interview with Dr. Tomiko Tawaraga, then head of the Office of Medical Devices in the Evaluation and Licensing Division within PFSB, MHLW, on January 17, 2008). By January 2008, some were still under review, and others were approved but awaiting a decision on reimbursement; still others were under pre-clinical trial consultation or under consultation for submission. These efforts are also part of an industrial policy that has received increasing attention since then: to fund domestic companies and to encourage them to develop new products and bring them to market.

The candidates for fast-track approval needed to meet three criteria: (i) offer a medical benefit to patients suffering from a life-threatening disease; (ii) have a major impact on the daily living of patients suffering from a life-threatening disease; and (iii) provide a treatment for diseases for which treatments were not yet available in Japan. After thirteen devices were selected, MHLW asked the industry—Japanese and foreign alike—to submit applications for highly needed medical devices. The candidates that survived this step-by-step process were submitted to a fast-track review and approval process. A final step consisted in identifying cooperating companies that not only had the wherewithal to develop these much-needed medical devices, but that also had the necessary clinical data.

Efforts at closing the "drug lag" made progress, but it was not clear whether these steps would really help close the "device lag." An industry insider felt that while MHLW recognized the "device lag," it simply took some of the products in the queuing line and put them ahead of the devices in the queuing line (Interview #35). This description can be interpreted in two ways. First, it illustrates that whatever well-intentioned efforts MHLW engages in, business circles will never appreciate them; they are impatient. Second, these short-term steps are necessary to modernize regulation and have better outcomes in the medium and long term. Realistically, very little is to be expected in the short term.

MHLW moved along several fronts simultaneously, adhering to a regulatory framework committed to the trio of the "quality, efficacy, and safety" of medical devices (PMDA, 2010). Yet these terms are ambiguous. American and EU documents in recent years use the term "effectiveness" rather than "efficacy." This is because: "the term 'efficacy' refers to the impact of a technology on health outcomes under ideal conditions, and 'effectiveness' refers to the impact of a technology on health outcomes under general or routine conditions. Common usage of this distinction is relatively recent" (Lewin Group, 2002: 54, footnote 10). Official Japanese documents perpetuate a myth of "efficacy," which realistically can only be achieved when health technology assessment capabilities are in place.

The leadership of MHLW, acting under pressure from the Cabinet Office in December 2008, instructed PMDA to speed up the regulatory process. In response, PMDA not only announced several measures but also implemented them through a cluster of regulatory tools to be carried out in stages. In the first stage, medical devices were categorized into three groups based on novelty: "new medical devices," "improved devices," and "me-too" predicate medical devices (similar to the US 510(k)-approved devices). MHLW and PMDA planned for a three-track review system based on the novelty of the medical device in 2011. Review procedures were standardized and review criteria and guidelines developed. Specialist review teams were to begin reviews of different groups of medical devices. Strategic collaboration with academia and PMDA, including exchanges with foreign universities and research centers and other relevant organizations, was to deliver the missing expertise that could not be secured by hiring from the private sector. Training methods of the US FDA and review organizations were to serve as learning tools. All measures for testing drugs and medical devices were to use the NIH measures as reference (UNDESA et al., 2012: 40). All initiatives are clearly medium- and long-term solutions. The number of reviewers was expected to increase further by 2013.

A second regulatory tool was introduced. PMDA was to run an initial evaluation system for new medical devices and perform a pre-application review of data. Relevant data include biological safety testing, electrical safety testing, and performance testing. Approval criteria and review guidelines were established, distinguishing between medical devices that require clinical study data and those that do not require them. PMDA was shooting for a reduction of the application review time of around seven months for new devices and four months for already developed or "me-too" devices. The goal for the review time was set at ten months. If no clinical data needed to be submitted, the goal for the review time was set at six months. The record of median total review time for medical devices, both for priority review products (to close the device gap) and for standard review products, improved slightly (PMDA, 2010: 24) and further improved by 2013 (National Policy Unit, 2012; UNDESA, ESCAP, ILO, UNEP, 2012).

History seems to repeat itself. Progress is made only in response to external pressures. In the mid- and late 1980s, as a result of tremendous pressures by the US government on the Japanese government in the so-called MOSS talks, the Japanese had agreed to a review time of twelve months for new medical devices, four months for "me-too" devices, eighteen months for drugs, and six months for IVDs. The current text is almost identical to that of the text from twenty years ago.

A third measure was to increase the number of consultations. My sources reported that MHLW and PMDA were inefficient and unhelpful; at the same time, MHLW complained that device companies sponsoring clinical trials did not make good use of the consultation options. PMDA is now expected to improve all of its consultations concerning market approval and clinical trials, and to clarify procedures and standards to be applied. The number of clinical trial consultations for medical devices and IVDs went up from a low of 29 in 2005 to 104 in 2009, and for IVDs from a low of one pre-clinical consultation to 6 in 2009 (PMDA: 2010: 24). These measures are designed to introduce predictability of document and data submission requirements *ex ante*.

In the future, PMDA was expected to devote all its energy and resources to reviewing the higher-risk Class III and IV medical devices. This was made possible by delegating the reviews of Class II devices to a third-party certification body rather than PMDA. Japan emulated the European Union's *new and global approach* to market approval, which puts so-called notified bodies in charge of reviewing and CE-marking medical devices to certify conformity with the essential requirements in EU law. A predictable by-product of this move to third-party certification is the presence of global consulting firms in Japan, like Emergo, BSI, and TÜV. In 2012, TÜV acquired twelve certification bodies around the globe and planned to do the same in 2013 (*Süddeutsche Zeitung*, June 26, 2013).

A fourth regulatory tool was designed to improve the audits by PMDA. Then PMDA conducted conformity audits covering GLP, GCP, GPSP inspections, and data reliability assessments. In reality, reliability assessments were primarily document-based goods inspections. Inspections increased from one in 2005 to 890 in 2010 post-marketing study practice (GPSP). Other tasks included the reexamination or reevaluation of clinical data compliance with good laboratory practice and good clinical practice. GLP inspections increased from 2 in 2005 to 8 in 2009, GCP inspections from zero to one in 2009. GPSP increased from 82 in 2006 to 107 in 2007, though it decreased to 65 in 2009. PMDA conducts on-site and document-based inspections of sites that require a license from MHLW and "appropriate manufacturing facilities (GMP/QMS)." Inspections rose from 4 in 2005 to 66 inspections in 2009, and from 0 to 3 in 2009 for IVDs (PMDA, 2010: 25).

Finally, PMDA also carried out GCP inspections. In conducting GCP inspections, PMDA inspectors also gave first-hand advice to the physicians, pharmacists, and nurses at the medical institutions to improve the clinical trial environment in Japan (PMDA, 2010: 25). Whether the 2010 report of PMDA reflects a well-intended program for future action, and whether the conduct of clinical trials in medical institutions actually improved, is hard to tell and should be an item on a future research agenda. The same is true for the two government reports published in 2012.

All activities are intended to speed up the closing of the "device lag," but they also need to be seen against the backdrop of increasing domestic conflicts and competitive pressures among US companies, which they export abroad to compete for and gain increasing market shares in Japan and elsewhere. This tension is visible not only in the competition between the orthopedic and cardiovascular product sectors, but also among the cardiovascular device companies themselves. During field research in Tokyo in 2007 and 2008, there was a frenzy over three products: the Cypher by Johnson & Johnson,[2] the DES by Medtronic, and the Taxus by Boston Scientific. The battle among the three device companies was over which stent performed better and had more permanent and satisfactory outcomes: the bare-metal, drug-eluting, or drug-coated stent? A related issue was how they should be classified: as a new medical device or a "me-too" device? Classification determines reimbursement and the kinds of review and approval processes for market approval. Further discussion of the superior performance of the three types of stent is referred to the *Lancet*, a London-based medical journal, which published a meta-analysis of the literature on the subject (Stettler et al., 2007: 937–948).

Morbidity and mortality data in Japan show that cardiovascular diseases are on the rise (WHO, 2010: 139–140). Cardiovascular diseases were the second highest diseases in terms of frequency in Japan, and cardiologists expected the morbidity rate for cardiovascular diseases to rise in the future (Kondo, 2007). An interesting question, then, is who is pushing and who is pulling for stents: doctors, business interests, or both?

One company insider spoke to the dominant role of doctors (Interview #7). Drug-eluting stents (DES) can be beneficial, but whether they are effective depends on the type of patient. There is no across-the-board answer for all patients. DES is a breakthrough device, and patients benefit from it. But cardiologists choose the method to treat a particular health problem, and on this basis they opt for the type of stent they will use. Until March 2007, only the Cypher by Johnson & Johnson was on the market, and J&J faced no competition (Interview #7). Then Boston Scientific came along with the Taxus stent for use in long coronary lesions. Today, three manufacturers are on the Japanese market.

The burdens for getting approval of stents are unevenly distributed. The first applicant has the hardest time to overcome all bureaucratic hurdles (Interview #7). A "new medical device" requires pre-clinical testing and clinical testing (Interview #7). The Johnson & Johnson Cypher received authorization for three years. Boston Scientific submitted the Taxus as a "me-too" device and accepted the "me-too price"; that is, a lower reimbursement rate. After three years, a reevaluation is scheduled and J&J must resubmit an application. Then MHLW can impose new conditions and mandate that, for example, strict and costly post-market surveillance measures must be carried out for the next three years, that a clinical trial with a definite number of patients must be conducted, etc. Johnson & Johnson enrolled two thousand patients for the Cypher (Interview #7).

Why are similar innovations treated differently? Is this narrative an illustration of regulatory arbitrariness and lack of rationality on the part of Japanese bureaucrats, or does it reflect the conventional wisdom behind regulating "me-too" devices on the basis of a predicate technology? The FDA applies this approach to the so-called 510(k) notification, and the EU approach tolerates a similarly lax method for allowing high-risk devices on the EU market. This era of lax passage of high-risk devices may be over. As previously mentioned, the United States and the EU respectively have debated related reforms since 2010, but no solutions are finalized as yet.

"Japan has few developmental capabilities, and there is no way we can compete," said Dr. Huimin Wang, MD, the Tokyo-based corporate vice-president for Japanese and Intercontinental Divisions at Edwards Lifesciences, Ltd. "If America is the elephant of the industry, then Japan must be compared to a dog or a cat" (Wang, 2005: 1–4). In Japan, the industry has been successful in moving the agenda forward and getting something done, but it has been less successful in preventing periodic cuts in reimbursement levels and low price setting, which accentuates the medical technology gap in Japan. In reality, business with medical devices is a lucrative business, and growth rates outpace those of other industrial sectors worldwide (Table 8.1). Yet complaints about burdensome regulations are heard in all venues that matter for regulatory affairs globally (Emergo, 2011). Reporting in the *New York Times* (November 5, 2009), Barry Meier published data that show the profit margins of the leading global device makers whose voice was heard loudest in Japan.

Table 8.1. Operating profit margins.

Zimmer: artificial hips and knees	30.0%
Medtronic:* heart devices, spinal implants, stents	28.6%
St. Jude Medical: heart devices, pain treatment devices	25.8%
Stryker: artificial hips and knees	23.1%
Boston Scientific:** heart devices, stents, diagnostics	23.1%

Source: Barry Meier. *The New York Times*, November 5, 2009. Credit Suisse, the original source, estimates based on company records.
*Includes other expenses
**Excludes amortization

"Success Is 70 Percent Cultural and 30 Percent Technical"

"Success is 70 percent cultural and 30 percent technical" was the conclusion that a regulatory affairs professional with Boston Scientific drew after having gone through a complex review process post-PAL, with a combination product, a Class IV (high risk) (Brizmohun, 2008: 16–18). Cultural and linguistic problems easily lend themselves to misunderstandings and must be differentiated from the complexity of laws, enforcement tools, and standard operating procedures (SOPs), including the intentions and motivations of the Japanese bureaucracy. Brad Hossak, a US-based American expert, as reported by Brizmohun (2008: 16–18), gave several recommendations to his American peers:

> Allow local staff to "wordsmith" into Japanese phrasing and give them editorial freedom.
> [. . .]
> Japan is a wonderfully perfectionist society and any typographical, translation and cross-reference errors will slow the final approval process.
> [. . .]
> It takes up to six months to receive permission to conduct a Japanese clinical trial (instead of some days in Europe and the US).[3]
> [. . .]
> A company should delegate all of its negotiations to local Japanese staff and answer inquiries within a two to four week period.
> [. . .]
> Don't get caught in the headquarters' "signature" process when too many executives want to sign off on the responses to the regulator.
> [. . .]
> Use local medical physicians to review the answers . . . and the STED should be updated accordingly. (2008: 16–17)

Along similar lines, Dr. Tomiko Tawaragi, then the director of the Office of Medical Devices of MHLW, in 2006 advised US companies, "*Improve communication between Japan office and US head office!* and *Communicate with the reviewers at PMDA*" (Tawaragi, 2006, slide 3, underlined in original). Ames Gross, president of PBM, advises American executives and salespeople how to think and move in foreign cultures. His firm advises on how to manage Asian cultural diversity and human resources issues, like recruiting, retention, and training (Gross, June 2005: 77).

Culture and Regulatory Science

In this context, the reader should remember the lessons from legal scholarship on the reluctance of Japanese officials and individuals alike to release health-related information (Higuchi, 2007c, 2007d, and 2005). Culture and privacy legislation is interlinked, and cultural influences are certainly at work in rulemaking and rule application concerning medical devices in what is called a "straitjacket society" (Miyamoto, 1994).

In the theory of regulatory science, clinical trials for drugs and high-risk medical devices are an integral and indispensable part of the approval process for market authorization in Japan, as they are in other countries (MHLW/Clinical Trial Issue Review Committee [CTIRC], 2006). In practice, physician-led clinical trials of medical devices in Japan were rare and only recently became the topic of serious discussions. MHLW officials complained that companies sponsoring clinical trials did not make good use of clinical trial/pre-application consultations.[4] Companies insisted on the absence of guidance by MHLW and the backward structural conditions in research development, medicine, and clinical research.

Under ideal circumstances, a clinical trial should involve an academic scientist, from the design of the study, through all its phases, until completion. Dr. Toshiyoshi Tominaga, speaking for MHLW at the *HBD West Meeting* on January 11, 2007, in Durham, North Carolina, said, "Investigators and subjects have few incentives to carry out or participate in clinical trials in Japan." In addition, he said, "The infrastructure is insufficient" and the capacities for medical device clinical trials in Japan are "slow, of low quality, and expensive." As a consequence, sponsors are "reluctant" to do clinical trials in Japan, and there is "too much dependence on foreign development." Moreover, "R&D is smaller" in Japan than elsewhere. He seemed less certain whether an alleged "lack of capacities" existed. Rather, Dr. Tominaga saw an "unfortunate vicious cycle" at work (Tominaga, 2007).

Although the weakness of Japanese universities as research centers for basic research was known in the early 1980s (Broida, 1982: 83–99) and continues today, the MHLW only launched a "Clinical Trial Promotion 3-Year Plan" (2003–2005) and a "Clinical Trial Promotion 5-Year Action Plan" (2007–2012) and invested 1.1 billion yen in "Research Grants for Clinical Study Infrastructure" in 2006. According to Tatara and Okamoto, "Clinical epidemiology in Japan is still poorly developed and its contribution to evidence-based medicine research worldwide regrettably small" (2009: 78).

Creating Innovation Capabilities

Innovation 25 was a report drafted in the Cabinet Office. In his first term in office, Prime Minister Shinzo Abe appointed Professor Kiyoshi Kurokawa to serve as the special science adviser to the Japanese government. He was the former president of the Japanese Science

Council of Japan and a member of the government Council for Science and Technology Policy. He was trained as a kidney specialist and taught and practiced medicine in the United States and Japan. He was also known as an outspoken critic of Japanese universities. What is best for Japan's research and development efforts? His answer was, "First you have to reform the leading universities" (*Science*, 2007: 186).

The aim of *Innovation 25* and the *Five-Year Strategy for the Creation of Innovative Drugs and Medical Devices* (part of *Innovation 25*), like the improvement of the regulatory side, was to bring the Japanese industry on board in an effort to make medicine and the medical device industry a driving force of developing world-leading products (*Five-Year Strategy for Innovation Creation and Medical Devices*, 2007), in direct response to global pressures (Finn, 2010b). Both initiatives were an integral part of a strategy to upgrade the drug sector internationally, but they also created benefits for the medical device sector (*Five-Year Strategy for Innovation Creation and Medical Devices*, 2007; the Prime Minister and His Cabinet, 2007).[5]

The original Five-Year Strategy pursued three objectives. A first objective was to obtain intensive research funding and increase a drug/medical device-related budget; to set up coordination units for industry, government, and university priority development areas; and to improve and consolidate the R&D tax system. The second objective was to nurture venture firms by increasing research funding, sharing facilities and equipment, establishing a corporatization support framework, using former players, improving advisory services, and discussing subsidy of user fees. The third objective was devoted to the improvement of the research and clinical infrastructure, including the promotion of multinational clinical trials, training personnel to assist physicians in clinical studies, and taking actions to improve the assessment of clinical performance of physicians. A regular public-private dialogue and stronger coordination between the relevant ministries, research institutions, and industry were to secure its success.

In April 2007, MEXT, MHLW, and METI, under political pressure from the Cabinet Office, were instructed to endorse the five-year strategy despite a long history of jurisdictional and ideological disputes among them. For the three ministries seemingly to move into an interagency mode of communication and cooperation was seen by several sources as quite unusual (from the nonscientific side, Interview #18, Interview #22, Interview #29, and Interview #62; from the scientific medical community, Interview #12 and Interview #32). The interviewees all agreed that without the leadership of Prime Minister Koizumi and his successor, Prime Minister Abe, and without the pressure of the Cabinet Office on MHLW, METI, and MEXT, this cooperation would not have materialized. However, by the time I conducted the interviews in Tokyo in 2007, it was already clear that the Koizumi reforms fell short of their promises.

In the past, the Ministry of Health was said to have had a firm grip over the local industry and even indirectly on the Japanese trade associations. This hold was facilitated by the phenomenon of dispatching retired bureaucratic elites to the twenty trade associations to influence their agenda (Interview #57) and keep an effective liaison with MHLW. The phenomenon is known as *amakudari* or "descending from heaven." The idea behind the expression is that former high-level civil servants, upon retirement, are switching over to executive positions in the private sector. Through the JFMDA, MHLW influenced local branches of device companies via the circuits established by this traditional practice. Foreign companies allegedly opposed MHLW, but domestic companies had no choice but to buckle under and accept the ministry's commands (Interview #35). By 2006 and 2007, attitudes had changed, and policymakers engaged in a different strategy.

Three Japanese experts (Interview #57a, Interview #57b, Interview #57c) with long-term experience in medical technology affairs at the JFMDA asserted that cooperation between the industry and the Ministry of Health then and now did not mean the same thing. In the old days, there was no communication between them and MHLW at all; today they talk. Moreover, while Japanese companies once were almost completely oriented toward the domestic market, they have now begun to export to the American and European markets (Interview #57a). Yet the sources left no doubt that government people are very influential still (Interview #57a, Interview #57b, Interview #57c), despite the recent changes—political, communicative, and behavioral.

What Is Government/MHLW Policy, and What Are Its Politics?

The elements of regulatory policy are known, as are the past tensions and contemporary turf battles between METI and MHLW. From the perspective of MHLW officials, METI is meddling with jurisdictional issues and control by MHLW over Japan's national health insurance program and the delivery of health care. On the other hand, METI is seen to show a willingness to move forward, understand the market, and allow business to be active (Interview #35). METI's authority and political capital stem from three sources: it has authority over the pharmaceutical industry and clinical trials of drugs, it is a fierce advocate of market-oriented private health-care solutions, and it is in charge of information technology. All three factors are significant challenges, directly and indirectly, to the authority of MHLW. METI has moved the pharmaceutical sector into new modes of operation and into the era of global competition (Schaede, 2008: 239–243). The government now intends similar developments for the medical technology sector (National Policy Unit, 2012).

Who is ultimately in charge—METI, MHLW, the Cabinet Office, or committees attached to METI, MHLW, or the Cabinet Office? The answer is difficult to determine. A source explained that medical technology companies working through ACCJ feel that they cannot afford to alienate MHLW, which they need for their device approvals, by siding too openly with METI (Interview #23). An academic expert close to the Cabinet Office spoke of a "miserable" state of affairs in clinical research and development (Interview #62). It was not clear whether the expert was referring to the weakness of the clinical and research infrastructures or the determination of Japanese device makers to specialize in diagnostic medical devices to the exclusion of treatment medical devices, or to both.

On the other hand, two Japanese academic observers (Interview #29a and Interview #29b) were not proud of the government's approach to promote medical-technological innovative capabilities, improve the clinical infrastructures, and advance medicine in Japan. They doubted that Japanese companies would ever become more active in this field. As proof, they made clear that leading firms such as Mitsubishi or Toshiba did not participate in these initiatives. In the past, the government contracted out too much to second-rate, quasi-governmental research organizations (Interview #29b), and not to top researchers.

The characterization of a three-party turf battle—between MHLW, METI, and MEXT—inferred from fieldwork contrasts slightly with the view that sees MHLW in full control of regulatory and reimbursement matters (Campbell and Ikegami, 1998; Ikegami at MTLF, 2007). In an interview on May 2, 2007, with Professor Naohiro Yashiro, who also attended the *Leadership Dialogue*, he explained that he agreed with Professor Naoki Ikegami on 90 percent of the issues and disagreed with him on 10 percent. Whether this disagreement stems from the particular methodological approach in their respective research, their political beliefs, or their respective closeness to different power holders—Cabinet Office and METI or MHLW and *Chuikyo*—is difficult to make out. Professor Yashiro, an economist, works on macroeconomic issues associated with health care, and he promotes more market-based schemes under government supervision of a "managed market" (MTLF, 2007: 10). In contrast, Ikegami, a health policy analyst and expert in management, focuses on the meso/micro level of financing and funding health care, and he is a fervent defender of the Japanese health insurance system.

Medical Device Engineering Initiatives

The strategy outlined in *Innovation 25* seeks to pursue four objectives: (i) to improve access to drugs and medical technologies; (ii) to boost the domestic industry, which needs venture capital for innovation; (iii) to develop clinical infrastructure capabilities; and finally (iv) to train physicians and support staff. "Medical technology, in particular, is regarded as a strategic industry to focus on along with automotive, information technology and the environment for the future growth of Japan's economy," writes Yoshio Mitsumori, a medical device expert in Japan (2009: 1). According to AdvaMed-ACCJ, *Innovation 25* also aimed at better collaboration with foreign countries, notably with Asian countries and the United States, EU, and Canada. According to the five-year strategy document, "The present system for evaluation of medical devices will be reviewed by consulting the industry concerned to increase the incentive for development and commercialization of new medical devices in harmony with the sustained availability of health insurance funds" (AdvaMed-ACCJ, 2007: 3). The language of *Innovation 25* is remarkable for its public recognition that the system is not up to par. Three official reasons were given for why Japan is pursuing a medical device industry vision now. To repeat, the first is a decline in international competitiveness; the second is an underdeveloped and inappropriate R&D environment in Japan; the third is to contain rising medical expenditures (Takakura, 2003).

Speaking for the JFMDA at the *Leadership Dialogue* in Karuizawa in April 2007, Mr. Wachi, then chairman of JFDMA and Terumo Inc., acknowledged that Japanese companies were lagging behind in medical-technological innovations (MTLF, 2007: 6). The industry suffers from and struggles under the constraining and ambivalent framework of

PAL. Elaborating on additional challenges faced by the industry and Japanese society, Mr. Wachi explained,

> The Japanese industry is growing, but 60 percent of medical devices are imported . . . The infrastructure remains very outdated. We hope that the Japanese industry will be revitalized through stimulation and competition with American companies . . . The Abe Administration is taking leadership, including introducing major new policies . . . However, the legal framework is still focused on a drug-oriented industry. But, we all know that drugs and devices are very different. For example, doctors or surgeons here are not able to use prototypes to test them and improve them. Simple changes require review from scratch. (MTLF, 2007: 6)

Japanese medical schools have departments for pharmacy but none for medical technology and science. This is in striking contrast to a total of seventy American universities that have medical device departments. Mr. Wachi explained that Japan only recently was "beginning to coordinate engineering and medical research. There is little training infrastructure and manufacturers have to pay for this training, but it is not reflected in final reimbursement" (MTLF, 2007: 6). A medical industry engineering consortium (METIS) also was established to coordinate the cooperation between industry, government, and academia to jointly set four goals: first, they identified seven areas for cooperation; second, with MHLW they intended to develop evaluation criteria for the next generation of medical devices; third, they worked on a proposal on how to improve clinical trials and clinical research; and finally, to improve the public's understanding of medical devices, more communication was needed.

Speaking on behalf of METIS, Hikaru Horiguchi, director of the Medical and Assistive Device Industries Office, presented METIS's vision on the promotion of R&D on medical devices, both in general and product-specific. For him the most urgent and essential task was to properly assess the social and economic values of medical devices (MTLF, 2007). In this context, seven working groups were organized around seven specific devices (implants, robotics, gene therapy, etc.) that are expected to become available in Japan on a large scale. These groups met monthly to discuss how to implement this medical industry engineering initiative, and how to bring medical and engineering science and industry practice closer together. They also discussed an array of regulatory issues, and how and what to report to METIS. JFMDA paid for these meetings (Interview #28).

Members of the working groups were recruited either from academia or the industry. While few of the academic members were experts in the engineering sciences, most of the remaining members were physicians. This raises two fundamental problems. There is a clash between available academic knowledge and the knowledge and the applied skills needed for the design and development of medical devices, including the servicing of IT and medical equipment, once high-tech equipment is installed and used in health facilities. For example, clinical engineers rather than physicians service heart-lung machines, artificial respirators, or defibrillators. The absence of physicists or engineers on the staff of hospitals is unacceptable to the industry (Interview #28). In his view, any improvement in designing, developing, and bringing medical devices to market was a long-term project of between ten to twenty years (Interview #28). While career opportunities did not exist in 2007, it is unclear whether any have been created through the various measures of the *Five-Year Strategy*.

All initiatives can be seen from two different perspectives. One perspective draws attention to a well-documented tradition of protectionism in Japan, and this argument was heard from foreign observers. They implied that *Innovation 25* and the *Five-Year Strategy for Creation of Innovative Drugs and Medical Devices* were nothing more than evidence of Japan's protectionist tradition. To impose strict regulations serves as a pretext to gain time until the domestic industry is up to snuff and ready to compete with the US-based industry. A second interpretation denies any such potential of the Japanese industry. To recognize an industrial vision and to design a strategy to accomplish it is one thing; to implement the vision and the strategy is an entirely different one. Japanese contacts saw implementation as *the* problem; they felt that these initiatives do too little and are too late (Interview #28; Interview #29; Interview #23; Interview #57).

How successful is this politically inspired, interagency collaboration among the three ministries? Interviewed contacts saw a good deal of rhetoric and symbolism in the statements in *Innovation 25* and the *Five-Year Strategy*. They did not see the statements as evidence that serious efforts will be made to invest in R&D or that resources will be made available. From interview sources, two additional paradoxes in Japanese public life can be inferred that shed light on the clash between a normative vision, reality, and perception of reality in Japan. A leading member of one of the seven committees to work on innovation creation in Japan felt that once people establish a program or follow a strategy, they have a stake in the success of the program and the strategy (Interview #28). The government, the bureaucracy, and even members of academia pretend that the measures are successful, when in fact they fall short of it (Interview #28). If you read the report of METI, he explained, you get the impression that METI runs a successful program. But officials and staff in METI are known not to spend much time on medical technology development (Interview #28). The outside observer can only draw one conclusion: medical technology innovation is hardly among METI's priorities.

The second puzzle refers to the link between product development, pre-market evaluation, and clinical tests (Interview #28). A first stage in development is or should be an evaluation of the design of the product. If the results are good, one can move on to manufacturing the product. Two major hurdles exist. The first is related to missing expertise among the company staff. Usually, the staff working on regulation in a company pays attention to the permission process, has good experience in tough negotiations with government people, and knows how to simplify the process by cutting through bureaucratic stumbling blocks. However, they do not have the experience to discuss clinical studies and clinical evaluations, which are essential to the development of new medical products (Interview #28). And this is what they ought to know in order to navigate the submission process.

The other hurdle is PAL. Accordingly, a manufacturer cannot set up such an evaluation system and will not get information on the performance of a device through an *ex ante* clinical evaluation. If a medical device company cannot begin a development with an evaluation—now called clinical evaluation—it cannot exist as a medical device company (Interview #28). PAL reversed a logical order: the authorization process comes first; meeting the requirements for GCP comes second. But starting the authorization process hardly gives confidence in a particular protocol or design. How do companies get the clinical evaluation that is needed for the authorization stage (Interview #28)? PAL mentions GCP, but PAL considerably changed its content and meaning and created a catch-22 situation. The industry insider explained that his company never had done clinical evaluations with patients before; prior to 2004, it did clinical evaluations in cooperation with a hospital on the basis of a procedure, but even this system was ambivalent and unclear (Interview #28). Whether the new law approved in 2013 (PMDL), and its separate chapter designed for medical devices, will resolve these issues in the future remains to be seen.

The committee advising METI (chaired by my source) decided to take up clinical evaluation and clinical studies and bring it to the attention of the government (Interview #28). The committee had thirteen meetings with government officials. Asked about the results, he felt that in general the discussions were useful, but also frustrating. All along, the government officials pretended that Japan pursued the same regulatory approach as the US FDA (Interview #28). At that time Japan only aspired to emulate the approach of the FDA's Center for Devices and Radiological Health; it was a goal for the medium and long term. Japan eventually will have "an investigational evaluation system, a fast-track program and a more comprehensive consultation system" (Mitsumori, 2008: 1). Japan did not have it in 2007.

The staff responsible for design in his company (Interview #28) suggested contacting the Institutional Review Board (IRB) of a hospital for a clinical evaluation, like in the United States. In the United States, the rules are well established, but they are not the same in Japan. Nobody knows the legal boundaries, and no one knows when you overstep them (Interview #28). While PAL came out of the blue, it had far-reaching consequences for device makers and the industry.

Finally, I wanted clarification about the alleged traditional but hidden protectionism at work in these initiatives and programs. In one of my last interviews in Tokyo, on January 17, 2008, I put this question squarely to Dr. Tomiko Tawaragi, then the director of the Office of Medical Devices within PFSB (MHLW). While she did not take issue with the question, she responded, "Most of the new devices are US-manufactured products. And the Japanese government's emphasis on highly needed medical devices benefits the US industry too." However, a close look at the list of selected devices revealed that many Japanese products in 2008 were on the list. In any event, over the last few years the Office for Medical Device Evaluation and the Economic Affairs Division inside MHLW must have had a challenging job in balancing the books and reversing a twenty-year-old practice of prioritizing cost containment over the need for advanced medicine and treatments.

To explore whether the original objectives and the new measures of the *Five-Year Strategy*, added in 2012, have been able to not only stop but also reverse the "vicious cycle" in clinical infrastructure and clinical research capabilities should be on a future research agenda.

In summary, this chapter demonstrated how and why the Japanese government engaged in the promotion of medical technologies, infrastructure investment, and the commercialization of medical products. Even if this round of reform measures is successful, and new and advanced medical technologies reach Japanese patients much faster than in the past, it will take considerably more time, effort, and resources before Japanese patients' access to modern treatments is comparable to patients' access in the United States and EU. Chapter 9 will address the problems that have to be resolved first; that is, meeting the requirements of GCP, reporting adverse events, funding medical research, and improving cardiovascular medicine.

Notes

1. The copy of this report was obtained from Professor Kiyoshi Kurakawa, MD, special adviser to Prime Minister Abe, at the interview with him on May 10, 2007.
2. Johnson & Johnson also produces bare-metal stents, in addition to drug-coated ones.
3. One or two days for obtaining permission to start a clinical trial seems overly optimistic.
4. In 1997, two tools concerning foreign clinical trials were available. The first was entitled "On Data from Clinical Trials of Medical Devices Conducted Overseas," specified in MHW/PAB Notification No. 476, March 31, 1997; the second carried the title "On Clinical Trials of Medical Devices Conducted Overseas" (MHLW/PFS/Notification No. 0331006, March 31, 2006) and was followed by Q&A interpreting the notification. In 2005, the enforcement tool "Ministerial Ordinance: Good Clinical Practice for Medical Devices" was issued (MHLW Ordinance No. 36 of 2005). Guidance on good manufacturing practices was issued in 1997.
5. Although medical devices are part of the strategy, the text primarily speaks to a new drug vision and by implication, a new medical device vision. The above text is verbatim from a figure entitled "Basic Concept of Drug Industry Policies: Deliver world-leading drugs and medical devices to the nation and drug/medical device industry to be Japan's growth-leader."

9

Realities of Clinical Medicine

Previous chapters reviewed medical technology regulation and recent government initiatives to close the "device lag" and analyzed the difficulties of bringing innovative products and medical technologies to the Japanese market. Whereas the introduction, diffusion, and use of medical technologies present challenges everywhere (Cohen and Hanf, 2004), the "device lag" and market difficulties are uniquely problematic in Japan. This chapter will address the enforcement and implementation of good clinical practice (GCP) and adverse event reporting (AER) as mandated by PAL, from a variety of perspectives—domestic and international, professional and administrative—in addition to drawing on the experience of Japanese sources, e-newsletters, and secondary literature. The aim is to demonstrate how and why the two legally mandated building blocks of PAL—in reality, borrowed from the international STED—cannot be implemented immediately, given the existing clinical conditions in Japan, and to show why the "device gap" (that is, inferior evaluation and review capabilities) will continue for some time to come. PAL has had profound implications for sponsors of clinical trials and for doctors and hospitals (Eno, 2006).[1]

Obstacles: First-Order and Second-Order Problems

A number of first-order and second-order problems hinder rapid improvements of clinical realities, capabilities, and advanced medicine. For one, first-order issues are those associated with PAL, a one-size-fits-all legal framework for drug and medical devices with its dominant drug orientation. Second, the health bureaucracy initially did not provide sound medical device-specific guidance to device companies. Finally, all measures to improve the clinical research environment start from a low level of support, with little, if any, political backup from the JMA or support by political actors with clout. A solution to the first problem is in store. The Pharmaceutical and

Medical Device Law was approved in late 2013 and will be implemented in 2014 and over time.

Second-order problem areas are multilayered and deeply entrenched in Japanese society, culture, and attitudes. In April 2007, Dr. Yukio Matsutani, the director general of the MHLW-Health Policy Bureau, presented the problem clusters that the HPB had prioritized for reform as follows:

- To ensure public trust in medicine,
- To maintain a quality system,
- To secure access to health care information and formulating new health care programs by individual prefectures (i.e., regionalization and [the new approach favored by health policy reformers]),
- To assure safety in health care delivery,
- To engage in a parallel approach of health care system reform along with infrastructure reform for innovative medical technology development and application,
- To promote clinical trial revitalization in a five-year plan,
- To promote medical institutions and clinical researchers collaborating in clinical trials, etc. (2007: 5–6)

This huge agenda has several problem clusters. Each cluster is complex in itself and requites skilled resources and much patience. Taken together, major efforts are necessary to resolve them satisfactorily in the medium and long term.

Universal Issues and Issues Unique to Japan

This catalogue of second-order problems with their multiple layers and changeable combinations forms the context conditions for enforcement and implementation of GCP and AER. Both originate in global harmonization efforts through ISO 14155, an international standard covering medical device clinical investigation, broadly defined (Giroud, 2009).[2] Global misunderstandings of ISO 14155 and GCP have both modified and amplified the interpretation of GCP in practice. ISO 14155—the international standards—was further amended and became ISO/FDIS 14155 in late 2010 (Kenny, 2010a; Stark, 2011). ISO 14155 and GCP are international norms that medical device and drug companies should follow for pre-market regulatory requirements and post-market clinical studies (understood as non-regulatory). For experts there are subtle differences between ISO 14155 and GCP. How each is implemented, in large part, depends on the clinical infrastructure capabilities in a country.

The Confusing Language of Good Clinical Practice (GCP)

All medical device regulatory regimes include the prescription of good clinical practice (regulatory) as a core building block covering regulatory requirements for clinical data, which are needed for market approval (pre-market phase) and non-regulatory studies (post-market clinical investigations) (GHTF, 2007). The Japanese medical device GCP uses similar language as the international version, but a twofold linguistic and analytical problem makes the GCP in Japan exceedingly complex. First, the new rules governing GCP for medical devices, including diagnostic products, in Japan are even more inspired by pharmaceutical standards than anywhere else (Azuma and Iseki, 2012); and second, the requirements for dossier submission were written with drug dossier submission in mind. Clarification of the medical device-specific dossier submission requirements only came with the so-called submission workshop in November 2006 (AdvaMed, 2006) and may have further improved since then.

The rules on the GCP consist of several layers: compulsory or legally binding mandates and standards, and voluntary or optional guidelines. Standards include ISO standards, Japanese Industrial Standards (JIS), standards set by the global Harmonization Task Force, and the like. PAL requires that the MHLW specify the certification and approval standards and the review guidelines.

A new medical device GCP standard took effect on April 1, 2009, and new reporting requirements for Institutional Review Boards (IRBs) came into force a year later.[3] Following the publication of a draft in October 2012, new medical device-specific instructions may become available in 2013 and later. The interview data exposed individual problem clusters and facets of the world of medical device GCP that, taken together, paint a rather discouraging picture of the GCP environment.

Prior to 2005, the GCP required a minimum of sixty patients (thirty patients each at two sites). A Japanese expert explained to an English-speaking audience that "the new GCP has no minimum and now requires the number of patients, which statistically proves its efficacy. In addition, the newer GCP requires strict monitoring to ensure that cases are being conducted in a proper manner. The new GCP basically conforms to the International Conference on Harmonization standard (for drugs) and is similar to requirements of the US FDA" (Mitsumori, 2006b, 26–28).

According to an official source (MHLW/CTRIC, 2006), an international multi-site clinical trial requires the participation of one hundred to two hundred Japanese patients. Practice seems to diverge from official policy.

An expert from the ortho world, in an interview on May 28, 2007, doubted whether even the practice prior to 2005 ever made any sense. What good is a clinical trial with sixty patients in a one- to two-year period when the objectives of a hip implant are durability and longevity (Interview #35)? Orthopedic implants are very successful and have been approved and used for twenty years in Europe and the United States without any requirement of clinical data. Spending a few million dollars on clinical trials is not justified. The market for orthopedic products is split into ever-smaller market segments—for example, implants for men and women, or orthopedic implants for Western patients and Asian patients (Interview #35).

In contrast, Japanese scientific experts with a medical or pharma background totally disagree. A clinical trial with patients from only two hospitals is unscientific and violates any methodological requirements for testing drugs (Interview #6; Interview #12; Interview #32). For them, the method used for testing drugs is the only valid scientific method. What they fundamentally object to is the absence of placebos and control groups—"the gold standard" for testing drugs and IVDs internationally. Professor Marc F. Swiontkowski, a surgeon and physician, explained, "Control groups and placebos are totally irrelevant for an implanted artificial heart" (2007: 12). This is difficult to swallow for pharmacologists and seems to have been a major problem for medical device approvals. "Surgical procedures are not pills" (Swiontkowski, 2007: 12). At the same time, to withhold surgery from a patient who is suffering from a heart attack is not an option. Surgeons must respond fast, and they need a rapid response to the evolution of complex systems. To test heart implants, Swiontkowski advocated multi-center clinical trials, but he was fully aware that these would raise "international issues" (2007: 12). By the same token, the late medical technology expert Clifford Goodman insisted that "the traditional evidence principles" and "hierarchies" designed for pharmaceuticals originally are inappropriate for a good many medical devices (2000). Cohen and Hanf also offer a realistic appraisal of medical device clinical practice (2004: 157–164).

The Root Causes of Current GCP Practices

The practices prior to PAL are traceable to the activities conducted by the Pharmaceutical and Medical Devices Evaluation Center (PMDEC), which was established as part of the National Institutes of Health Sciences (NIHS) in mid-1997. PMDEC served as research center under MHW (predecessor of MHLW). At that time, the center had no specific medical device reviewers at all. In September 1998, PMDEC recruited three medical reviewers with clinical experience and three medical device officers with administrative experience. Yasuhiro Fujiwara's account of cancer drug clinical trials is discouraging:

> In contrast to the FDA, there are no open-to-the public detailed criteria for anticancer drug approval in Japan. However, there exists a guideline describing how to conduct clinical trials for an anticancer drug, but it is out of date. New Japanese approval criteria, such as "approval requirements, off-label usage, oral anticancer drugs, noncytotoxic anticancer drugs, and proposal for clinicians" are only now being developed. (Fujiwara, 1998: 7–19)

The Japanese format and language—not necessarily the substance— follows the international language. Seven criteria are spelled out and must be followed: (i) specifications; (ii) *stability and durability* (italics in original); (iii) conformity to the criteria specified under Article 41, Paragraph 3 of PAL; (iv) performance; (v) risk analysis; (vi) manufacturing methods; and finally (vii) results of clinical studies (Matsumura, 2006; MHLW/CTRIC, 2006). Obviously, items (i) through (vii) have different implications for testing drugs and medical devices. For example, stability and durability of a drug is scientifically different from stability and durability of a medical device implant.

Features Unique to Japan

In 2002, the MHLW introduced "The Three-Year National Drug Clinical Trial Action Plan," which pursued five strategic areas: (i) promoting clinical trial networks; (ii) enhancing clinical study systems within medical institutions (including the training of twenty-five hundred new clinical research coordinators); (iii) supporting patient enrollment in clinical studies; (iv) reducing burdens imposed on the pharmaceutical industry; and finally (v) advancing and promoting overall clinical research (MHLW/CTIRC, 2006).

The Global GCP Compliance Report 2006: US, EU, and Japan reports a few weaknesses unique to Japan (Barnett Educational Services, 2006). Like the United States and the EU, Japan adopted the ICH's Good Clinical Practice Consolidated Guidelines in 1996, implemented the guidelines, and applied them to drugs through complex sets of ordinances and notifications. In 2004 in Japan, these GCP standards were expanded for the first time to cover medical devices. Sponsor responsibilities and standards for medical institutions, IRBs, and clinical investigators were identical. The new rules also laid down the conditions for study monitoring and audits (Barnett Educational Services, 2005: 193–206).

While Japan's long-standing reluctance to accept foreign clinical data has been a hot topic on the US-Japan agenda for quite some time, this issue was resolved in part in 2007 when MHLW began to accept foreign clinical data, provided that the medical device trials were conducted in conformance with the Japanese equivalent or superior standards. The MHLW failed to present a clear idea of what actually could be validated through clinical trial testing of medical devices, claimed a scientist (Interview #32), at least until fairly recently.

Japan expert Yoshio Mitsumori told a devastating story:

> Many queries raised by PMDA do not coincide with the guidelines set forth by the country's ministry of health. . . . PMDA has been too slow to initiate actual evaluation; for example, orthopedic implants take eight months on average before a review takes place. Even standardized medical devices take too much time to review, and non-standardized medical devices are much worse. . . . Evaluation can be slowed or even reset due to a change of the reviewer in charge. Basic skills and/or knowledge about particular medical devices by specialty often are lacking to cope with a wide variety of products and new technology coming to market. (2009b: 1)

Overall management of device evaluation has been poor.

Medical Device Clinical Studies

In theory, MHLW accepts clinical trials that are conducted following the American medical device GCP regulation and are accepted by the US FDA. Tomiko Tawaragi (2006), then medical device chief within MHLW, explained that MHLW was committed to a policy "to accept foreign clinical data to the greatest extent possible." In practice, the real problem is that clinical trials for medical devices must also be compatible with the Japanese GCP that follows the logic of the drug GCP (Fukui, 2001: 626). In 2006, the Medical Device Evaluation and Licensing Office in Japan clarified, "When a medical device has been approved in the US (or is being examined for approval) and is submitted in Japan, it is recommended that a complete set of efficacy, safety, and performance data of the product that was submitted to the US

FDA be also submitted to the Japanese counterpart from the outset" (AdvaMed, 2008: slide 12). The practice of following the drug GCP continued in 2012 (Azuma and Iseki, 2012).

The problems with medical device clinical studies are compounded by the underdeveloped clinical trial infrastructure (Kakizoe, 2008: 8). There are several problems. First are the questions of what clinical evidence is needed for market approval *ex ante*, how much is expected of clinical studies *ex post,* and how this is differentiated for drugs versus medical devices. This may seem like a set of easy questions, but even with international definitions increasingly provided by GHTF working groups, regulatory authorities have different interpretations, resulting in the persistence of divergent national regulatory practices. Moreover, what is accepted as clinical evidence for drugs and medical devices is not necessarily the same to Japanese, American, or European pharmaceutical or medical device experts.

Other issues that still need to be resolved on the international and domestic levels are the length of study periods, the number of study sites and subjects per application, and the kind of clinical trials (that is, open, non-controlled trials or mostly controlled clinical trials). To repeat, there are only "few medical institutions with proven performance in medical device clinical trials" (MHLW/CTIRC, 2006).

Japan is unique even among Asian countries, according to Ames Gross and Caroline Tran. They write,

> The most important thing to understand regarding clinical trials in Japan is that few things are set in stone. The exact number of test subjects and trial sites is subject to the interpretation of the examining office of the MHLW, and varies with each product and examiner. Decisions on a company's clinical trials can vary widely, depending on which MHLW examiner is consulted, his or her mood, and other subjective factors. Different examiners may recommend vastly different numbers of case studies for exactly the same product. After giving a preliminary opinion, the same examiner may arrive at a completely different conclusion days later. Or he or she may decide that more studies are needed, even if no new information is presented. (Gross and Tran, 2002)

In theory and in practice, hard evidence about the safety, performance, and efficacy of medical devices comes from *ex post* clinical studies, which more often than not are performed in uncontrolled environments. PMDA approves a medical device, a distributor sells it to the hospital, and PMDA decides on the facilities with physicians who are sufficiently trained to conduct them. Said one contact, one never knows where a device ends up in what part of the country (Interview #15).

Jurisdictional Issues

A second problem cluster refers to jurisdictional issues, which are best characterized as conflicts between the Safety Division (MHLW) and the Ministry of Education (MEXT). When complaints about PMS and clinical studies, conducted in line with the letter of the law, are reported to the Safety Division (MHLW), the division cannot intervene in clinical studies (Interview #37). MEXT has this responsibility and determines and controls the budgets of university hospitals in consultation with MHLW. University hospitals are national hospitals participating in the national health insurance program controlled by MHLW. As explained by two sources (Interview #37, Interview #57), if complaints about PMS and clinical studies are raised, the issue needs to be resolved between the Ministry of Education and a national hospital. If a product defect or a human error is involved, it will have to be resolved both between a clinician and the company and between the clinician and the hospital. MHLW can only get involved in cases where the welfare of patients in all of the eight or nine regions in Japan is in jeopardy.

Members of an advisory committee can recommend the recall of a product. Then the Safety Division (MHLW) has to weigh carefully what countermeasures to take and what clinical evidence to request, explained an MHLW official (Interview #37). The division wants clinical evidence, but clinical studies will take a very long time, and they are costly. Device makers take a short-term view and want a decision right away. After an incident with a medical device is reported, the division has to find out first who was in charge and who carried out the safety measures, and then clarify the legal issues. If MHLW acts on the recommendation of a review panel to recall a product that later turns out to have been faulty, the Japanese will blame the MHLW in their "culture of blame" (Interview #37).

The Global Compliance Report 2006 reveals another factor unique to the PMDA in Japan compared to other regulatory agencies in the United States and Europe.

> There are several factors that make profiling Japan's evolving GCP compliance program a particular challenge at this point. Among these factors are the subtle, yet significant, differences in the authorities

and responsibilities of Japan's PMDA compared to regulatory agencies in other countries. The PMDA, for example, does not have the authority to undertake direct inspections of clinical investigators or IRBs, only to confirm the quality/GCP compliance of data that were submitted in marketing applications through "reviews" of source data and other documents at sponsor and institution (clinical investigator and IRB) facilities. Such subtleties make it difficult for those familiar with other regulatory systems to understand Japan's GCP compliance system, those close to the process warn. (Barnett Educational Services, 2006: 195–196)[4]

Lack of Trained Physicians to Carry Out Clinical Studies

A third problem is the lack of trained physicians to do clinical studies. Only a few doctors have had an opportunity to do a clinical trial (Interview #15, Interview #32, Interview #48, Interview #12, Interview #55). Japan lacks medical specialists. In the past, no training in how to conduct clinical research was offered. And training in a specialty is relatively new. Japan has more than eighty medical schools, of which forty-two are national medical schools subject to the Ministry of Education, eight to local government, twenty-nine private, and one military (Hirao, 2007). Physicians are not interested in R&D or in conducting clinical trials. New graduates seem to choose training at university hospitals, but "they tend to seek training in small departments like ophthalmology, dermatology and plastic surgery" (Hirao, 2007). The number of residents choosing internal medicine, surgery, and pediatrics is relatively low. In short, Japanese doctors train to become general practitioners and to treat patients as primary-care physicians (Muraoka, 2005).

Medical specialty training was first mandated only in 2005, and specialty boards, as they are known abroad, do not exist in Japan. Continuing medical education (CME) was enacted in 2004. It is a first step in the direction of eventually offering refresher courses. Based on the written evidence (Ikegami and Campbell, 2008; Rodwin, 2011a) and the interviews, one conclusion is self-evident: the JMA has had no interest in standardizing medical procedures in medical specialties. Japanese medicine clearly is lagging behind medicine in other advanced societies.

A fourth issue is the lack of appropriate incentives to engage in a clinical trial. Young physicians perceive serving as a principal investigator in a clinical trial as not helpful for their professional career path (Interview #15). Publications count more than hands-on skills in surgery (Minami, 2004). Japanese clinicians should engage in clinical research themselves instead of reviewing old studies done in Australia ten years earlier that may no longer be relevant (Interview #15). Getting reputable clinicians engaged in clinical studies remains a serious issue. Gross and Tran (2002: 3) explained,

> Until recently, clinical trials were considered taboo in Japanese culture: physicians who participated in them were often stigmatized. This has created a huge barrier for clinical trial testing in Japan. In recent, years, however, there are emerging initiatives, in the forms of TV commercials and informational Web sites, to better educate the Japanese public about the merits of clinical trials.

Younger clinicians begin to recognize that cooperating in a clinical trial is becoming more valuable for an academic career (Interview #15).

Patient Recruitment

Patient recruitment for clinical trials presents a fifth problem (Interview #12; Interview #15; Interview #51); it is a difficult job that takes time and patience. Japanese patients have universal access to doctors through the national health insurance program. They trust their doctors and hold them in high esteem; they do not question them, but they do not receive information about available treatments from them either (Interview#12; Interview #51). Getting their informed consent is even harder, costly, and an almost impossible task (Interview #12 and Interview #51). Legal scholarship agrees with this assessment (Higuchi, 2007c and 2007d).

The High Cost of Clinical Trials in Japan

A sixth problem is the excessively high cost of clinical research and getting clinical data. Maintaining a clinical research infrastructure is an expensive proposition everywhere, but the costs for clinical trials in Japan are excessively high. They are reportedly twice as high in Japan than in the EU and the United States (MHLW/CTIRC, 2006: 41). The *ACCJournal* asserted in 2007 that clinical trials in Japan cost twice as much as in the United States and ten times as much as in South Korea (*ACCJournal*, 2007: 19). The contributing factors are lengthy bureaucratic review and approval processes, repeat negotiations with MHLW, repeat consultations with PMDA over the proper protocol for clinical trials, and the high cost for using a mandatory market authorization holder (MAH) (L. E. K. analysis,

2005). High living costs and the high cost of doing business in Japan should be added.

How and whether compensation is paid by a company in Japan depends entirely on the arrangements between the hospital and the company (Interview #12, Interview#15). An investigator has a budget but does not have money. Every dollar goes to the hospital (Interview #12). How doctors enroll patients depends on the physician's contract with the hospital (Interview #15). The issue of patient compensation for participating in clinical trials is contentious in Japan, as in other countries.

Ethics Committees

A seventh problem is ethics committees. These do not work the same way in Japan as elsewhere (Interview #17; Interview #51: Interview #61; Eaton and Kennedy, 2007). Ethics committees were established on a voluntary basis starting in the 1980s; by 1992, all medical schools were reported to have initiated ethics committees. The regulations on institutional review boards (IRBs) did not exist until 2008. In the meantime, each institution did its own thing (Interview #12; Interview #51; Interview #32; Interview #48). What rules are applied? I put this question to Professor Akabayashi, a renowned specialist in medical ethics in the Department of Biomedical Ethics within the Division of Health Sciences and Nursing at the Graduate School of Medicine of Tokyo, in an interview on January 30, 2008. He has written widely on ethics and medicine in Japan (Akabayashi et al., 2007: 1–9). According to Akabayashi, the committee in part goes by its own internal rules and in part follows rules established by the FDA and the National Institute of Medicine (2001). As chair of the ethics and IRB committees at the University of Tokyo medical school's hospital, he added that the IRB predominantly deals with clinical drugs and, to a lesser extent, with medical devices. Unfortunately, he had no specific statistics to share.

For him, conflict-of-interest issues fall into three categories of relationships that need consideration: (i) university hospital/investigator, (ii) investigator/patient, and (iii) investigator/industry relations. He values the patient-investigator relationship the most, but the others are significant as well. A statute on the relationship of industry and investigator did not exist, but with the increasing attention to the medical device manufacturing sector, Japanese officials may develop a separate statute for it.

The design issues concerning medical device clinical trials were fundamentally not so different between the United States and Japan, according to Professor Arakawa of Tokyo Medical and Dental University Hospital. But one difference exists and concerns the endpoints of clinical trials. In osteoporosis, for example, the FDA considers the endpoint to be a bone fracture. By contrast, Japan used to consider bone (mineral) density to be the endpoint; it changed to the FDA classification a few years ago. Because placebos also raise ethical issues and risks, particularly over a long period of time, they would not go forward in Japan (Arakawa, 2005, 2006a, 2006b, 2006c; Arakawa and Omata, 2003).

Under these circumstances, it is ludicrous to expect Japanese medical specialists to be the drivers of medical-technological innovation. The continued, albeit lessening, split between scientifically oriented clinicians at a few top medical centers and the majority of physicians, who are physician owners of hospitals, clinics, and laboratories, is not helpful for any progress. Physicians and physician owners benefit from a legacy of privilege and have too much to lose. The "uneven axis of power" (Ikegami and Campbell, 2008: 107) not only hurts the objectives of medical technology regulation and patients' access to advanced treatments, but it also damages the innovative capabilities of Japanese device companies. Despite a few initiatives (reviewed in Chapter 8), the stumbling blocks to modernization of the regulatory apparatus and the clinical infrastructures, and advanced treatments to Japanese patients, are a legacy of weak or nonexistent clinical capabilities combined with a strong state tradition that has failed to promote a strong medical technology tradition and advanced medicine.

A few local initiatives may eventually improve clinical capabilities in Japan. For example, the University Hospital of the University of Tokyo's Medical School entered into an alliance with seven major hospitals, called the University Hospital Clinical Trial Alliance (UHCT Alliance). Participating hospitals developed standardized application forms, informed consent forms, and procedures to be used by all UHCT Alliance members as a model on a voluntary basis.[5] The manuals and "ideal models" were developed in cooperation with an interdisciplinary team lead by Professor Akabayashi. Considerable progress has been made by the UHTC Alliance over the last five years (Matsumoto et al, 2013). The revised *Five-Year Strategy of 2012* mentions the importance of such initiatives, calling them essential for moving forward.

Every small hospital wants to do heart surgery, regardless of the skill level and experience of its surgeon. Doing heart surgery is attractive to patients and hospitals; for the former it brings relief of suffering or death, and for the latter it brings revenues. Complementing Rodwin's account (2011a: 184–203) and confirming Minami's personal experience (2005), four contacts (two close to industry, a hospital manager, and a cardiologist) felt that the salesperson in some instances had more knowledge than the doctor (Interview #43, Interview #55, Interview #36, Interview #15). At times it would even be dangerous if the salesperson was not in the surgical room. Close contacts between a device company and a surgeon are also seen as limiting the competition among surgeons but strengthening the position of the physician-owners of hospitals instead. Such contacts are typically shrouded in secrecy everywhere. Another background variable stands out. In 2007, about six thousand private practitioners were owners of clinics or hospital in Japan out of a total of ninety-five hundred, and they negotiate individual deals with each company. For the remaining thirty-five hundred hospitals (including university hospitals, national hospitals, and municipal hospitals), different conditions exist, and negotiations are conducted at a higher level of government.

An Unhealthy Research Climate

Several key witnesses to scientific medicine spoke to an unhealthy professional research climate in universities in Japan (Interview #32; Interview #51; Interview #55; Interview #14). In their view, even research-oriented clinicians do not and cannot openly discuss their research findings with colleagues. How do Japanese doctors get information about new medical technologies and innovations? Obviously Japan does not enjoy the same level and abundance of information available in the United States, according to one scientist (Interview #32). In his view, the *New England Journal of Medicine*, the *Lancet*, and even the *New York Times* health section are good sources of information for those who read English, but most Japanese doctors do not speak or read English. Attending international conferences is another means of learning about new developments. Getting training in a foreign medical institution is another option. Finally, he explained that US companies have made abundant information about their products available in the last few years (Interview #32); sometimes it is the only information on medical innovations in Japan.

Reporting Adverse Events (*Hiyari Hatto*)

As with GCP, Adverse Event Reporting (AER) is a vital, normative, and empirical building block of medical technology regulation on a global scale. AER focuses on product-related incidents to the exclusion of incidents related to medical or human errors. Japan PAL institutionalized mandatory requirements for reporting adverse events and near misses when medical devices are utilized. Reporting is mandatory for companies but voluntary for doctors. They should report when they suspect that a company might not report or when they become a witness of a near miss or incident. Failure to report violates PAL (Article 77-4-2), according to a field source (Interview #37).

Conceptually and analytically, AER is the policy instrument designed to secure efficiency, performance, and patient safety concerns. It marks the end stage in the life cycle of medical technology regulation and covers specific responsibilities, accountability, and transparency mechanisms. AER is a kind of litmus test for assessing whether risk regulation of medical technologies effectively institutionalizes patient safety concerns and whether device makers and doctors report such incidences (Eno, 2006, slides 5–11; Ishikawa, 2009: 1–13). Interest in patient safety, quality of care, and the Japanese health-care system is fairly recent. A "safety culture" needed to be developed from scratch, including the design of reporting tools and organizational changes in hospitals (Nakajima et al., 2005: 123–129).

What was the tipping point of this change? A major accident in a teaching hospital in 1999 culminated in the creation of a national reporting system that is in place today (Tominori Hasegawa, n.d.). As an expert in public health, Toshihiko Hasegawa (2007) argued that AER is an important responsibility in the interest of public health and for developing good statistics on the experience with the performance and outcomes of medical devices. Who communicated this important task to the respective audiences? This is difficult to determine. The same is true whether MHLW or MEXT offered special training for doctors and hospitals. JFMDA offered some training of safety officers in device firms.

Global Influences

Two factors, one global and one domestic, explain why the AER standards for reporting were revised in 2005. These underscore the increasingly dynamic interdependence between developments in Japan and abroad. The Global Harmonization Task Force and, in particular, Study Group 2 (SG2/GHTF) provided much international guidance on how to handle vigilance reporting or adverse event reporting in the medical device sector. Following such guidance, PAL mandated these changes in 2005 for drugs and medical devices. Whether the obligations for manufacturers and physicians are voluntary or mandatory is clearly a national matter. Prior to 2005, Japan worked with three categories of incidents: "serious," "moderate," and "mild," which are now replaced by the international differentiation between "serious" and "not serious" cases based on the work by the Study Group 2 (SG2/GHTF) and approved by the board of GHTF.[6] The so-called global harmonization model originally came from the European Union.

Flexibility is built into the global model. In Japan, "serious" incidences that result in death are distinguished from "serious" incidences "other than death." Incidences involving death must be reported within fifteen days, and "serious" ones must be reported within thirty days. While the reports are shared among the regulatory authorities and the industry, they are off limits to researchers, doctors, and patients. In other words, the communities that ought to know something about risks, recalled products, and the negative results of clinical trials of medical implants, for example, know next to nothing about the causes of an incident, the recall of a device, or the results of clinical trials.

Overall Control, but a Division of Labor

The responsibilities for medical technology regulation and the regulation of health-care institutions and health professionals are tightly integrated within MHLW. The Safety Division within the Pharmaceutical and Food Safety Bureau (PFSB) is responsible for adverse events with drugs and medical devices, while the Health Policy Bureau (HPB) is responsible for medical and human errors. HPB receives the information on adverse events via the Japan Council for Quality Health Care, established in 1995 and a non-profit organization funded by the Japanese government; the JMA; and other health-care-related associations (Toshihiko Hasegawa, 2007, 2002). The Japan Council for Quality Health Care (JCQHC) serves as contact for the reporting by hospitals and doctors. It collects and analyzes all reports before they go to the MHLW, the PFSB, and the Health Policy Bureau. The database in regard to medical products, device failures, or comparative performance data is slim (Tatara and Okamoto, 2009: 136). How could it be otherwise, when "doctor's malpractice has seldom been sanctioned provided that the case remains a civil dispute, and calls for something to be done about 'repeaters' of such malpractice have become more intense" (Tatara and Okamoto, 2009: 136)? One thing is clear: as long as prevalence data on AER assembled by the Health Policy Bureau are not integrated with the prevalence data on medical errors, little is really known about risks and harm to patients.

Reporting Behavior

From a very low level of reporting in 1996, the reporting of AER to MHLW/PMDA by companies shows an ascending curve over a ten-year period; by contrast, the rate of voluntary reporting by physicians (based on PAL) is excessively modest at any time period (Table 9.1). A revision of stricter reporting obligations for doctors and hospitals was

Table 9.1. Medical devices and adverse event reporting.

Fiscal year	Medical device companies reports	Medical device companies (foreign reports)	Medical professionals	Total	Research reports
1996	119	-	2	121	13
1997	240	-	56	296	17
1998	445	-	76	521	10
1999	555	-	88	643	13
2000	2,749	-	173	2,922	18
2001	5,026	-	166	5,252	21
2002	5,026	-	266	5,252	54
2003	5,013	-	370	5,383	38
2004	11,515	4,210	622	16,347	157
2005	6,222	5,012	445	12,152	37
2006	9,310	2,880	424		
2007	13,842	2,708	434	17,156	
2008	4,301	2,014	444	6,759	
2009	4,116	2,332	363	6,811	

Source for the period of 1996 to 2005: Hideo Eno, deputy director, Safety Division, PFSB, MHLW. 2007 (received May 2007). I interviewed him on May 30, 2007. Available from: http://www.pmda.go.jp/English.reports.html. The data from 2007 through 2009 are from PMDA, *Profiles of Services Fiscal Year 2010*, p. 28, available from: http://www.pmda.go.jp/english/html (accessed 10/28/2010). Information on research reports for the years 2007 through 2009 are not available. Moreover, company reports submitted until FY 2003 include foreign reports. Why there is such a dramatic drop in reports from device companies in 2004 and 2005 and again in 2008 and 2009 is unknown.

not anticipated in 2007 and 2008 (Eno, 2006: slides 2, 5, 25, and 42). An undiminished influence of physician-generalists and the JMA vis-à-vis the MHLW could be at work. If the JMA "does not oversee licensing or conduct professional discipline," writes Rodwin (2011a: 200), and if "significantly the MHLW disciplinary committee is not proactive" and "lacks investigative powers and relies on reports of misconduct brought to its attention," they have no incentive to report. Why would they report? Nakajima, Kurata, and Takeda (2005: 114–117) have studied the reporting of adverse events and confirm the lack of a reporting culture.

The Medical Care Act

What PAL failed to do by not mandating health-care providers to report, the Medical Care Act was meant to accomplish (Tatara and Okamoto, 2009: 114–117). The Medical Care Act (also known as clinical practice law or medical practitioners' law) was amended in June 2006 and entered into force on April 1, 2007. It ordered the creation of a safety system in health care at all medical institutions and the establishment of medical safety support centers at all prefectures and cities with public health centers (Tatara and Okamoto, 2009: 47). On paper it looks like an ambitious plan, but the Medical Care Act only ordered hospital management to appoint a designated AER staff member. In small hospitals, this responsibility is carried out by the same individual who is in charge of drugs and medical devices. And in large hospitals, AER reporting is divided between two individuals: one is responsible for the reports on incidents or near misses with drugs, the other for medical devices. Retailers and MAH license holders have a similar responsibility. PAL and the Medical Care Act have institutionalized AER. But AER is only as good as long as someone monitors, verifies, and takes action in case of an incident.

The "Revisions for the Reporting Standard of Adverse Events" singled out four groups of medical institutions for mandatory reporting, totaling 272 medical institutions. These include national advanced health-care centers and national Hansen's disease (leprosy) centers; hospitals set up by the national hospital organization; hospitals affiliated with universities under the School Education Law; and advanced treatment facilities (Eno, 2006; Tatara and Okamoto, 2009: 83–87). Other hospitals had the option to participate on a voluntary basis. In all, 533 hospitals out of a total of 9,070 hospitals in Japan participated in mandatory AER as of December 2005 (Tatara and Okamoto, 2009: 84). They reported about 1,063 events. In all, 278 hospitals voluntarily participated, and they reported 129 adverse events, which is an extremely low figure (Eno, 2006, slides 41–42). That these numbers reflect clinical reality is unbelievable.

If AER is the most critical tool to secure performance, efficiency, and safety in health care, the question arises: Why is only the public segment of all hospitals ordered to report? True, the mandate covers the large hospitals (533 in total, including the largest university hospitals), which have the highest number of beds. The continued legacy of what Ikegami and Campbell have astutely described as an "axis of power" (2008: 107), which includes physician-hospital owners, private hospitals, and for-profit hospitals, in addition to the JMA, probably hides an explanation. According to Rodwin, the JMA "has blocked the state and insurers from using utilization review, practice guidelines and other oversight" (2011a: 184). AER needs to be substantially improved (Nakajima et al., 2005).

"Off-Label Use" Revisited

In this context, it is worth returning to a discussion of the "off-label" use of technology by physicians and surgeons. An industry source (Interview #23) defended Japanese doctors, saying that they are pretty progressive and try out new therapies. They do not lack an interest in new ideas, but they need help. If scientifically oriented physicians had more political clout and influence, they could help the industry too. With the right political process in place, doctors would want to innovate. Japanese doctors use three-generation-old pacemakers. They are aware that even Chinese doctors are not in this situation; this is "a real travesty for them" (Interview #23). The reimbursement system is another reason why doctors cannot use the latest technology for treatments in Japan (Interview #23).

According to a Western-trained social scientist and consultant to Japanese hospitals (Interview #36), his team had spoken to many clinicians who openly admitted the desolate state of affairs but were too close to speak openly about it. Living in a very restricted space, they cannot speak up. Finally, he argued that the JMA was not a champion for excellence; instead, it was a big lobby that was interested in giving campaign contributions to politicians rather than in medical innovations.

Professional Liability

Doctors can do anything they want to treat their patients, commented a MHLW official (Interview #37). Like professional liability insurance in other countries, insurance does not cover the doctor if he or she uses a device for a purpose not authorized by the approval. Doctors, not device makers, are responsible for the consequences of "unauthorized use." Insurers have data on doctors' liability insurance and therefore on medical errors, but they won't release this information (Interview #37). Physicians are keen on doing the right thing, but they are nervous because they are now held responsible for medical errors (Interview #37). Accidents will occur, and then invariably people will blame the government and ask, "Why don't you restrict the doctors?" The government does not take any action (Interview #37).

Device makers have a simple answer. Incidents are not related to the products but to the skills of surgeons, other health-care providers, and the environment in which they are used (Interview #15). Companies try to obey the law and to report first, ask questions later. When the safety agency asks a company to present a solution to a problem associated with an adverse event, the company must have a solution in the first place. The regulator wants to know how the manufacturer intends to correct the problem. The US home office assured the Japanese branch office that the incident in question did not exceed the threshold of acceptable risk, a notion unknown to the Japanese. Instead, adverse events can mean many things, ranging from wrapping of a package being torn open (in the distribution chain or later in the health facility) to an adverse event while caring for a patient (Interview #15).

When the MHLW announced that doctors were expected to report directly to PMDA, device makers initially were concerned that they now would report every little thing (Interview #23). He conceded that the industry might have used this argument as an excuse and has been overprotective. Today, reporting is in place. Doctors report, and there are no problems (Interview #23). The data on AER are so crude and superficial that one can really doubt such an optimistic account.

Despite hurdles, in the last decade progress has been made, and more rationality has been introduced. In the 1980s, manufacturers would approach the US embassy for consultation and support, but nobody really had a handle on how to review and evaluate medical devices (Interview #20). There was a vacuum that an entrepreneurial doctor could fill. An anecdote illustrates the unlimited power of a doctor who also served in an official function. An ophthalmologist by training, and president of a small doctors' association and simultaneously a key political and professional player, he single-handedly reached the verdict that a particular product should not be allowed on the Japanese market.

No one dared contradict him: not a MHW official, fellow professionals, or members of the association. Change could only be expected after the doctor's death. In the 1980s, a single doctor, politically active, commanded a lot of clout (Interview #20). Did the foreign product in question compete with a domestic product? This question could not be verified in the field.

Funding of Medical Research

In 2001 and 2002, the government decided to establish six research centers to build a knowledge base in some specialties (Tatara and Okamoto, 2009: 79–80, 93–94).[7] I asked whether they qualify as centers of excellence, and two Japanese observers answered with a clear no. The concept "center of excellence" is missing in Japan (Interview #32; Interview #23; Interview #36). There are a few scientific societies, such as the Society of Oncologists and the Society of Cancer Therapy, that are not comparable to professional societies in other contexts. Scientifically oriented Japanese clinicians would never come to a device company with an idea of how to change a medical device, unlike their American and European colleagues (Interview #32; Interview #23).

MHLW is the funding agency for the six centers, and it has a small budget of about 6 million dollars to be granted to medical centers and hospitals around the country. In turn, the centers report to MHLW (Interview #32). Compared to the US NIH budget of some three billion dollars, the budget of these national research centers is modest. In addition to funding from MHLW, MEXT had a budget of some $1.2 billion for the life sciences at universities in 2006 (Ministry of Education, Culture, Sports, Science and Technology, 2006: 276).[8] Funds from METI are earmarked for basic research and technology, including information technology, and cannot be used for clinical trials (Interview #32). METI wants to fund private "seed" projects that are expected to grow into many activities to correct the backward state of affairs in the medical technology field. Despite a status quo-oriented structural environment overall, small, incremental steps toward enhancing the clinical research infrastructure and the clinical trial environment and promoting innovation capabilities are possible. The initiatives in cardiovascular medicine and heart clinical trials are small steps that seem to work.

Cardiovascular Medicine and Heart Clinical Trials

The US FDA and MHLW-PMDA have conducted joint discussions about cardiovascular medicine and heart clinical trials. The time from the conception of the idea to the first meeting in January 2007 took close to four years; since then, the two parties have met on a regular basis. The benefits from Harmonization-by-Doing (HBD) to the FDA and MHLW-PMDA are mutual. The United States and Japan face similar scientific issues, and safety and effectiveness issues are the same for the reviewers in each country. The ultimate objective of HBD is to develop common protocols that will lead to a list of well-known wishes.[9] "HBD works" was the enthusiastic response of Professor Yoshihiro Arakawa when I interviewed him about the HBD initiative on January 21, 2008 (Arakawa, 2007a). In addition to the US FDA and the Japanese MHLW, on the American side Dr. Krucoff and Dr. Jim Alexander, two cardiologists from Duke University, provide professional and entrepreneurial leadership. Professor Arakawa and Professor Sase have represented the Japanese academic scientific community since the beginning of the HBD initiatives, and they also represent Japan in international harmonization efforts through the GHTF, ICH, and ISO-related activities (Tawaragi, 2008).

No one doubts the usefulness of HBD. The industry is eager to sell drugs and medical devices, and cardiologists are ready to treat patients suffering from cardiovascular disease. Is the HBD project tilted in favor of US interests to move faster into the Japanese market? Having the two regulatory authorities and the stakeholders in one room to discuss a range of regulatory and sometimes controversial and scientific issues is preferable to behind-the-door discussions, especially when they talk to each other to avoid scandals; this is not acceptable, said one expert (Interview #32). And second, there must be an open agenda on the contradiction inherent in PAL and what it allows, and how the objectives of global harmonization will be resolved.

The HBD is uniquely committed to heart health, while the *Leadership Dialogue of Stakeholders and Policy Leaders* in Karuizawa, Japan, in April 2007 addressed broader questions of health-care problems in the two countries. To the extent that diseases were mentioned, the discussions focused almost exclusively on cardiovascular disease (ranking highest among the diseases in the United States). Cancer is the number-one cause of death in Japan. Joint replacements (hip or knee) for healthy people over age sixty-five received little attention. Several observations may explain why all attention was on heart health. First, it is an excessively complex issue for regulation, and it is the fastest-growing field in medical-technological innovation, with drug-eluting stents, implantable defibrillators, and pacemakers increasingly being used. Moreover, the tactics and strategies by the US heart device companies to gain access to markets and reimbursement on a global scale are fairly unique. A high-level executive is rumored to have authored what later circulated as white papers by AdvaMed and Eucomed. And representatives of the leading US heart device companies are increasingly active in international standardizations organizations. Second, the problem of the absence of drugs to treat cancer seems to be resolved. Cancer treatments are now available that only a few years ago were not. Pharma firms were restructured in Japan a few years earlier than the launching of the medical device industry vision (Schaede, 2008: 239–243). The efforts in the drug sector have borne fruit. Third, orthopedic devices for hip replacements are covered and reimbursed by the national health insurance program. They do not have to fight for a reimbursement code; they have one already.

In April 2007, American and Japanese conference participants, including cardiovascular and orthopedic surgeons as well as academic experts knowledgeable in the bioengineering world, were asked whether the 2007 *Leadership Dialogue* would change anything (MTLF, 2007: 23–25). Most American participants were skeptical that anything would change, but they acknowledged the goodwill of Japanese government officials for trying hard to be responsive to US concerns and complaints. It is possible that the conference was staged as a PR effort for the sole purpose of justifying the changes to come vis-à-vis many status-quo agents in Japan, in medicine, clinical practice, and in particular the organized Japanese medical profession.

By way of summary, the clinical realities on medical device clinical evaluation capabilities and adverse event reporting are broad in range and long term. In the last few years, modest progress on clarifying regulatory issues and building regulatory compliance has been made (PMDA, 2010: 28–32). Despite interagency collaboration and coordination among MHLW, METI, and MEXT launched by the government, the industry continues to view the *ex ante* and *ex post* controls as unusually burdensome in 2013. The "device lag" (delayed treatments) and the "device gap" (inferior evaluation capabilities) are not yet closed. Evaluation and review schemes for innovative medical devices are still inferior to those of the United States and the EU (Tan, 2013). Status-quo agents and the entrenched context conditions described throughout this monograph seriously impede the modernization of the regulatory project, the clinical research infrastructures, and the capability to engage in clinical studies and trials. And yet, modest progress has been made and is ongoing.

Notes

1. Pharmaceutical Affairs Law, Enforcement Ordinance and Enforcement Regulations, 2005/07. In October 2012, the MHLW published a first-draft proposal to revise the Ordinance of PAL and the Medical Device GCP (Azuma and Iseki, 2012).

2. As Danielle Giroud explains, "ISO 14155 does not intend to re-invent GCP. Rather it seeks to provide strong medical device-oriented guidance to an industry where many start-up companies have limited resources and regulators rightfully impose an increasing demand for clinical data both in the pre-market and post-market phases" (November 13, 2009).

3. The *Asia Medical eNewsletter* (2009) elaborates: The first change is regarding Institutional Review Boards (IRBs). Previously, medical institutions conducting clinical trials were obligated to set up and maintain their own IRBs internally, which can be expensive. With the new changes, a medical institution's director can designate an outside party to perform this task instead. The IRB must be part of a university, nonprofit company, or independent government agency, not a for-profit company. To preserve IRB transparency while making this change, the rules also add new reporting requirements. IRBs must make publicly available their internal procedures, members' names, and summaries of meeting minutes. The second change is regarding the physical handling of investigational products. Previously, the shipping of investigational devices and drugs (including confirmations of receipt and quality management) had to be performed directly by those running the clinical trial. Now, the trial sponsor can designate a third party to perform these tasks.

4. Editor's note: The PMDA prefers the term "reviews" to "inspections" in referring to document and on-site GCP assessments. Technically, only the MHLW has the authority to conduct "inspections," which it rarely does. But PMDA's *Profile of Services: Fiscal Year 2010* refers to "inspections."

5. The seven university hospitals are Gunma University Hospital, Shinshu University Hospital, Chiba University Hospital, Tsukuba University Hospital, Tokyo Medical and Dental University Hospital, and Niigata University Medical and Dental Hospital.

6. There is no simple definition of "serious" and "not serious" cases. The key elements are intensity and predictability of an injury or adverse event. The GHTF document *Medical Devices Post Market Surveillance: Global Guidance for Adverse Event Reporting* (SG2PDN54R6) describes "serious injury" (also known as serious deterioration in state of health) as either "life threatening illness or injury; permanent impairment of a body function or permanent damage to prevent permanent damage to a body structure; or a condition necessitating medical or surgical intervention to prevent permanent impairment of a body function when appropriate" (7). The document goes on to state, "The interpretation of the term 'serious' is not easy, and should be made in consultation with a medical practitioner when appropriate" (7).

7. The six centers are the National Cancer Center in Tokyo, the National Cardiovascular Center in Osaka (created thirty years ago), the National Center for Urology, the National Center for Children, National Center for Aging Health, and an international health center, the International Medical Center in Japan (IMCJ).

8. The table shows a budget of ¥282,453 million in fiscal year 2004 for METI, compared to a budget of ¥40,354 million at the disposal of MHLW.
9. "More robust clinical trials, improved clinical research infrastructure, better clinical data, better understanding of how the US and Japanese experience can complement one another, a new approach to early market availability of new treatment and devices to benefit patients in both countries, a mechanism to decrease lag time between US and Japanese product approval, an atmosphere of international collaboration between regulators, regulated industry, clinical researchers, patients and academia, a continuous progression in global harmonization" (US Food and Drug Administration 2011).

Summary and Concluding Comments

Who would have thought that Japanese patients have fewer chances to benefit from medical innovation than Americans and Europeans? The answer is hardly anybody. Most people in the West think of Japan as a technologically advanced society and as an equal to the United States and Europe. Why this is not the case in clinical medicine, clinical evaluation, and treatment capabilities of innovative medical devices in Japan, and how the government has responded to these conditions substantively, was the subject of this study. For a technologically advanced country like Japan, the discovery that medical technology, medical innovations, and clinical research were underdeveloped, and that patients had limited or delayed access to advanced treatments and procedures when compared to Europe and the United States, presents a number of paradoxes. This study sought to unravel them and go to their root causes so that I could explain how and why Japanese patients did not benefit from medical innovations like their European and American cousins. The study focused on medical device regulation during a period of dramatic changes, domestically and on a global scale. That domestic reform of an entrenched regulatory system moved slowly, and then only in response to pressures from an increasingly competitive international environment, is not unusual given the clash between rhetorical intent and actual implementation of regulatory policies.

Even at the conclusion of the study, some puzzles remain. A good many experts and scientists agree that over the years, Japan has made progress by increasing the efficiency of decision-making on devices, introducing some transparency into regulatory practices, and improving the review process. Despite considerable efforts to address these conditions in that period, the "medical device lag" and the "medical device gap" continue. In other words, the clinical procedures and treatments that are available to Europeans and Americans are not available in Japan, due in large part to inadequate clinical evaluation and inappropriate review capabilities and resources in Japan. Medical device professionals from various countries, and those associated with foreign and domestic companies, still describe compliance with Japanese medical device regulations as difficult and cumbersome, and Japan remains in a lonely position ahead of other nation-states.

This study of medical device regulation and innovation in Japan sought to identify the descriptive characteristics of regulatory authority and the context conditions surrounding the reform and modernization of the medical device regulatory framework in Japan that may help explain how reform and modernization yielded desired outcomes. Rather than accepting a dominant explanation that blames the bureaucracy and government for the delays in access to modern medicine and innovative medical devices, this study put forward a complementary, three-pronged proposition: first, that the Japanese medical profession had not transitioned to a modern profession, lacking the associated professional responsibilities and rights, including organization of its professional representation; second, that the medical technology sector historically has been a weak sector and one-sided with its focus on diagnostic medical devices; and third, that the government was unwilling to take on the powerful Japan Medical Association. Successive governments lacked the political will, even when they had the vision and leadership, to advance scientific medicine in Japan and make certain that the outcomes of clinical work and the latest medical know-how are available to Japanese patients under the umbrella of the national public health insurance program.

The Ministry of Health, Labor and Welfare (MHLW) and the Pharmaceutical and Medical Devices Agency (PMDA) have an important part in the "device lag" (when devices are not physically available) as well as in the "device gap" (when inferior evaluation and review schemes exist). On average, innovative medical devices are approved between three to five years later in Japan than in the European Union and the United States. Drawing on primary and secondary sources, interviews, and gray literature (industry newsletters, brochures, flyers, etc.), this study addressed the passage of the 2005 Pharmaceutical Affairs Law (PAL) and the external and internal environments surrounding it. PAL necessitated the writing of a huge number of implementing regulations, and in its aftermath it brought about a considerable number of significant institutional, legal, and organizational changes. A turning point came when the relationship between the relevant policy actors—the Cabinet or MHLW—was transformed and the political leadership instructed MHLW to move ahead more quickly in closing the "device gap," promoting medical innovation and medical science, and realizing the role of the medical device industry for economic growth in Japan.

At the heart of the debate about medical device regulation are the relationships connecting device companies and physicians to the government and bureaucracy, on the one hand, and the relationships connecting Japanese patients to the government and bureaucracy, on the other. There lies another profound contradiction among these relationships. This is the discrepancy between the power and influence of these three groups—the bureaucracy, the industry and individual device companies, and physicians—and the relative deprivation of patient access to the most innovative devices and procedures compared to their European and American counterparts. Japan is an unusual case where common assumptions are contradicted. For example, it has the highest number of heart specialists, but their training and (as Japanese experts have repeatedly pointed out) their specialty training and clinical experience do not measure up to the standards practiced in the West, and professional medical specialty organizations have been delayed. Only a segment of practicing specialists received postgraduate training, but they were certified as specialists. Moreover, the mandate for continuing medical education came late to Japan. In recent years, major efforts have been made to close the gap and catch up with specialists in other developed countries. Developments are moving forward in Japan, but change is coming slowly. Another example of a puzzle is that Japanese device makers are heavily invested in the diagnostic medical device sector, but they have stayed away from the treatment device sector. And last but not least, regulatory policymaking is a privilege of the executive branch and spurs interest-group politics and lobbying as well as academic and professional politics. However, the limited role of democratic politics and participation by the Japanese public remains intriguing.

In examining the core building blocks of medical device regulation, special attention was given to the factors that cause or facilitate institutional change and to structural power relationships between government, industry, and the Japanese medical profession at the heart of medical device regulation in Japan. Focusing on the domestic structures and on the historical pattern of ties and conflicts between the Japanese and American governments was critical to an understanding where

Japan was in the early 1990s, where it has been going since then, and how it was reforming and modernizing three underdeveloped areas: the medical device regulatory regime; clinical research infrastructures and clinical trial capacities; and entrepreneurship, innovation creation, and development.

The Medical Profession

The Japanese medical profession historically has generated enormous economic and political power and influence. The leadership of the Japan Medical Association (JMA) has been able not only to define and control its own work, income, and prestige, but also to extract from the bureaucracy compromises, deals, and bargains. This setup worked to the advantage of Japanese physicians, but at the same time one important side of a profession was shortchanged: namely the ability to define, develop, and control standards for all medical specialties rather than general medicine alone. This happened not simply because the JMA has ignored the issue, but also because the scientific medical communities—to the extent that some exist in a few specialities—have been too busy doing research for publication in the past, rather than engaging in developing medical standards. In the future, Japan needs more cooperation between scientists, academics, and clinicians; a reformed medical profession; and a reduced role in *Chuikyo* and its committees. Indeed, there is some evidence that the JMA seems to be well on its way to losing the grip it has had over its members—solo practitioners and physician-owners of hospitals—and its political clout.

The State, Government, Bureaucracy, and Manipulation

In much of the scholarship on the Japanese state and bureaucracy, it has been argued that foreign emulation and domestic continuity characterize politics and government in Japan. Yet the conventional interpretation of an interventionist state and an activist state did not provide any leadership or a vision for a weak medical technology sector in terms of manufacturing or medical-clinical capacities. The sector is heavily crowded with status-quo agents, strong veto players, and numerous professional castes. Neither the MHLW nor the JMA so far have signaled their readiness to break ranks in their long-standing and compromising alliance.

There also has been a debate about the classic tools of a civil service bureaucracy for retaining power and control: consultation, the role of advisory committees (*shingikai*), or the phenomenon of "descending from heaven" (*amakudari*)—that is, the placement of retired and previously higher civil servants as advisers to Japanese trade associations and large companies. Both work to protect and reinforce the interests of the ministries and government agencies. What is striking to a US-based observer is the Japanese preference of asking only academics to serve on committees along with businesspeople to the exclusion of a broader mix of individuals representing the public or different segments of civil society. Despite the ongoing transformation of public policy and the public sector since the 1980s, Japanese state institutions continue to yield undiminished influence and power in politics and policymaking. The bureaucratic elites have not been reluctant to reorganize institutions and to reform regulatory policy and public health policy, yet they have been unwilling to cede power and modernize the access that Japanese patients have to advanced medical treatments.

If the past is any indication, it is fairly unproblematic to put the blame for the weakness of the medical-technology sector on the Japanese bureaucracy and a lack of leadership, based on the well-known features characterizing the bureaucracy in Japan: bureaucratic self-interest, turf protection within strict hierarchies, and interagency rivalries, including close relations with the domestic industry on the one hand and with the Japanese medical profession on the other. The bureaucratic traditions in rulemaking and application and a legalistic and formalistic administrative culture tend to reinforce these characteristics. The legislature also bears responsibility for legislation and regulation, even when these are drafted by the civil service bureaucracy. Yet when challenged by foreign interests (the United States and the EU) starting in the late 1980s and throughout the 1990s, the Japanese bureaucracy has shown itself surprisingly responsive to such pressures within its constraints: budget constraints, priority given to cost-containment policies over closing the "device gap" and the "device lag," and bringing advanced treatments to Japanese patients, as well as the reform of the delivery of individual and institutional care.

The scheme to encourage innovation and launch a medical device industry vision focused on several initiatives, ranging from improving an R&D promotion tax and a device development project to a three-year national plan to revitalize clinical trials. When all is said and done, and despite what was said above, it seems that the bureaucracy is the only candidate that can turn ideas into reality and qualify for policy leadership, given the political culture in Japan. It may take time, but once the bureaucracy recognizes and diagnoses a need for change, regardless of from where the pressures for change are coming, it can act without much resistance from any group, including civil society. Instead of passionate political debates over the right balance between the interests of the industry, clinical investigators, and the general public, the study found accommodation, complicity, and many veto players with considerable political clout.

Between Symbolism, Enforcement, and Implementation

Given the paucity of applied research in Japan, it is difficult to always clearly differentiate those policy dimensions that fall into the category of symbolic policies from the policy goals and instruments that were meant to be enforced, complied with, and implemented. This research has had to make sense of policy statements formulated in flowery language and seemingly full of good intentions. But intentions are only as good as the resources made available to turn them into actual reforms. Since 2010, the Japanese government has given priority status to medical technology by creating a department within the Cabinet Office to enhance the competitiveness of Japan's medical business, including research, devices, and drugs. Yet Japan-watchers remain skeptical about policy declarations, particularly when no or few resources are made available to support policy intentions.

Change in a culture that is resistant to change is difficult to achieve, regardless of the circumstances and the policy sector. Occasionally, this may have led to overstating and overdrawing an argument; this is preferable to not engaging in applied research at all. It can be argued that the study is not as successful as it wished to be in clearly differentiating between the interaction effects of several driving forces: global market integration in medical goods and services, the dramatic technological and material innovations of the last twenty years that have improved the diagnostic and treatment capabilities of medical professionals, and an aging Japanese society that is no longer blindly trusting its doctors as in the past and is demanding more and better delivery of health care. The scarcity of English-language information and data hampers an understanding of medical technology regulation in all its various intertwined facets and the fluid boundaries between the analytical themes and related developments. Far from being a problem of language, it is also a lack of applied social science research in Japan.

Medicine and Technology

The rapid transformation of medicine over the last twenty years did bypass Japanese patients in a way. This does not mean that the major breakthroughs in medicine that occurred in several waves, decade after decade, in the twentieth and twenty-first centuries are not present in Japan. Ultrasound was introduced in medical applications in the early 1950s, followed by implantable pacemakers (1960s), CT scans (1972), and magnetic resonance imaging (MRI) and positron emission tomography (PET), both in 1977. The 1990s saw the addition of coronary artery stents, the improvement of laboratory testing, and new materials such as polymer in implants and fiber optics. These developments were so transformative that even the hardware makers and the world's leading trade associations felt it necessary to adjust their names to this new reality. For example, in the United States the Health Industry Manufacturers Association (HIMA) changed its name to Advanced Medical Technology Association (AdvaMed), while the European Confederation of Medical Devices Associations now is known as the European Medical Technology Industry Association (Eucomed).

In the last fifteen years, American and European spokespersons for the med-tech industry have been working hard, not to say aggressively, in all venues of influence and at all levels of multinational regulation, to convince payers and insurers of the value and benefits of health-care technology. They also have loudly complained about a multitude of obstacles in all health-care markets. Innovative and life-saving technologies can significantly contribute to cost containment. New technologies that improve quality of life (QOL) and independence for the aged are only possible in well-functioning markets that bring new technologies to patients in a timely and cost-effective manner. This point even still holds in Japan when devices are tailor-made for Japanese patients to fit them to the musculoskeletal system and lifestyle of most Asian patients. Both refrains are trumpeted around the globe. It may be true that free markets rather than "managed markets" can deliver medical-technological innovations faster to patient populations, but free health-care markets typically do not secure a basket of benefits, universal or close to universal health insurance coverage, and access to medical care independent of means and when needed. There is substantial body of cross-national literature on health-care reform that backs up this argument.

Global Harmonization

The breakup of the old Global Harmonization Task Force (GHTF) in March 2011 has no bearing on the interpretation of legislative and regulatory activities offered in this study. For eighteen years (1993 to 2011) the GHTF has brought together the Japanese regulatory authority and the med-tech industry with their counterparts from other GHTF founding member countries. Since 2011, the International Medical Device Regulatory Forum has taken its place, but without the participation of industry representation. Both the United States and the European Union have pushed for global harmonization and supported Japan's efforts to improve the overall conditions for medical technology regulation and developments and emulate a good many FDA or EU elements. Yet they have refrained from institutionalizing the STED or other vital parts in domestic law and regulation and instead continue to rely on their own traditional toolbox of regulation and domestic laws and actively engage in critically reviewing their respective regulatory regimes. The Japanese case offers a complementary narrative to any future narratives about medical technology regulation in other countries.

Over a period of approximately ten years the FDA relaxed its reluctance to third-party certification and even pressured Japan into adopting this approach for medium-risk devices. However, as this study demonstrates, transferring policy ideas from the United States, the EU, or the GHTF to the Japanese context does not occur in linear fashion. What works in the EU and the United States, and what is agreed upon at the global level, does not necessarily work in Japan, because of the substantial differences in institutional arrangements and tradition of public management and law. By the same token, what is agreed upon at the global level is not necessarily adopted nationally in very different contextual conditions. Embedded institutions, behavior patterns, and routines are among crucial root causes of slow development, many obstacles, and modest outcomes.

Bibliography

Abbott, Andrew. 1988. The *System of Professions: An Essay on the Division of Expert Labor*. Chicago: University of Chicago Press.

American Chamber of Commerce in Japan (ACCJ). 2006. The *ACCJ Business White Paper: "Working Together, Winning Together."* Tokyo, Japan: ACCJ.

———. 2001. *US-Japan Business White Paper*. Tokyo, Japan: ACCJ.

ACCJ Journal 44(11) (November 2007): 19–20. www.acjj.or.jp/documents_library

AdvaMed. 2007. *AdvaMed-ACCJ Joint Written Testimony*. Chuikyo Industry Hearing, October 24, 2007 (Courtesy Phil Agress).

———. 2006. *How to Comply with Japan's Regulatory Requirements: Strategies for Success*. Japan Submission Workshop, November 8–9. Tokyo, Japan.

———. 2005. *Bringing Innovation to Patient Care Worldwide*. http://www.advamed. org/publicdocs/PR-361.htm (accessed November 17, 2006).

———. 2008. *Action Program for Speedy Review of Medical Devices*. Revised December 11, 2008 (English translation of Japanese original, 2005).

———. 2005. "The New Market Authorization Holder (MAH) System for Medical Devices in Japan" (June). Published by AdvaMed.

Agress, Philip. 2006. "Regulatory Issues in Japan." Draft, courtesy Agress, AdvaMed.

Akabayashi, Akira, Brian T. Slingsby, Norko Nagao, Ichiro Kai, and Haime Sato. 2007. "An Eight-year Follow-up National Study of Medical School and General Hospital Ethics Committees in Japan." *BMC Medical Ethics* (June 29), 1–9. http://www.publicmedcentral.nih.gov.

Allsop, Judith, and Linda Mulcahy. 1996. *Regulating Medical Work: Formal and Informal Controls*. Buckingham: Open University Press.

Altenstetter, Christa. 2013. "US Perspectives on the EU Medical Device Approval System, and Lessons Learned from the United States." *The European Journal of Risk Regulation* (December 2013): 443–464.

———. 2012. "Medical Device Regulation in the European Union, Japan and the United States Commonalities, Differences and Challenges." *Steering Biomedicine: The Regulatory Dynamics of Therapeutic Technologies. Special Issue*, edited by Alex Faulkner, *Innovation—The European Journal of Social Science Research* 25(4): 362–388.

———. 2011. "Medical Device Regulation and Nanotechnologies: Determining the Role of Patient Safety Concerns in Policymaking." *Law & Policy* 33(2) (April): 227–255.

———. 2008. *Medical Devices: European Union Policymaking and the Implementation of Health and Patient Safety in France*. New Brunswick, NJ: Transaction Publishers.

Altenstetter, Christa, and Govin Permanand. 2007. "EU Regulation of Medical Devices and Pharmaceuticals in Comparative Perspective." *Review of Policy Research* 24 (5): 385–405.

Annas, George J., and Frances H. Miller. 1994. "The Empire of Death: How Culture and Economics Affect Informed Consent in the US, the UK, and Japan." *American Journal of Law & Medicine* 20(4): 357–394.

Arakawa, Yoshihiro. 2007. "Role of Academic and Government Leadership in Clinical Infrastructure—Japan Academic Perspective—How to Solve 'Speed and Cost' issues." Clinical Research Center, Tokyo University Hospital. HBD West Meeting, January 11 at Duke University, Durham, N.C.

———. 2006a. "About the Protocol Manual for Investigator-initiated Clinical Trials."Available at www.crc.u.-tokyo.ac.jp.index.html

———. 2006b. "Towards the Improvement of Clinical Trials." *Clinical Ethics* 4.

———. 2006c. "Specificity of Medical Devices Clinical Trial and the Assistance by the Clinical Research Center." *Clinical Engineering* 17 (3): 246–251.

———. 2005. "Key Issues in Support of Investigator-initiated Clinical Trials."*Rinsho Hyoka (Clinical Evaluation)* 32 (203): 505–512.

Arakawa, Yoshihiro, and Masao Omata. 2003. "Clinical Research Center of University of Tokyo Hospital for the Advancement of Clinical Trials: Towards the Highest Quality and Speedy Conduct of Clinical Trials." *Rinsho Hyoka (Clinical Evaluation)* 30: 2–3.

Asahi Shimbun, January 12–13, 2008. "Diet Enacts Relief Law for Hepatitis C Patients."

Asia Medical eNewsletter 9 (1) (December 4, 2009a). "Increased Cooperation between Japan, EU, and Canada for Medical Device Regulations." (http://www.pacificbridgemedical.com/newsletter/article.php?=440)

Asia Medical eNewsletter 9 (2) (February 2009). "Japan Releases Five-year Plan to Speed Medical Device Registration."

Asia Medical eNewsletter 9 (1) (January 2009). "Japan Revises GCP for Medical Devices and Drugs."

Azuma, Kentaro, and Hiroshi Iseki. 2012. "Analysis of Safety Reporting Requirements during Medical Device Clinical Trials in Japan." *Journal of Artificial Organs* I 10.1007/10047-013-0692-6.

Bartholomew, James R. 1989. *The Formation of Science in Japan: Building a Research Tradition*. New Haven, CT: Yale University Press.

Barnett Educational Services. 2006. *The Global GCP Compliance Report 2006: US, EU, and Japan*. Waltham, MA: Barnett Educational Services.

Battista, Renaldo N., H. David Banta, Egon Jonsson, Matthew Hodge, and Hellen Gelband. 1994. "Lessons from Eight Countries." *Health Policy* 30: 397–421.

Becker, Karen M. 2010. "Assessing the Proposed Changes of the US/FDA's 510(k) Programme." (September/October), www.regulatoryaffairs.medtech.com.

Bok, Derek. 1996. "Scientific Research and Technology." In *The State of the Nation*, 37–54. Cambridge, MA: Harvard University Press.

Brizmohun, Neena. 2008. "How to Avoid Approval Delays in Japan." *RAJ Devices* (January/February): 16–18.

Broida, Joel H. 1982. "Medical Technology in Japan." In *The Management of Health Care Technology in Nine Countries*, edited by H. David Banta and Kerry Britten Kemp, 83–99. New York: Springer.

Campbell, John Creighton. 1994. "Democracy and Bureaucracy in Japan." In *Democracy in Japan* (3rd ed.), edited by Takeshi Ishida and Ellis S. Krauss, 113–137. Pittsburgh, PA: University of Pittsburgh Press.

Campbell, John Creighton, and Naoki Ikegami. 2009. "Comprehensive Long-term Care in Japan and Germany: Policy Learning and Cross-national Comparison." In *Comparative Studies and the Politics of Modern Medical Care*, edited by Theodore R. Marmor, Kieke G. H. Okma, and Robert Freeman, 265–287, New Haven, CT: Yale University Press.

———. 1998. *The Art of Balance in Health Policy. Maintaining Japan's Low-Cost, Egalitarian System*. Cambridge, UK: Cambridge University Press.

Carpenter, Daniel. 2010. *Power and Regulation: Organizational Image and Pharmaceutical Regulation at the FDA*. Princeton, NJ: Princeton University Press.

Clinica (1299) (March 21, 2008).

Clinical Trial Issue Review Committee (CTIRC). *Clinical Trial Issue Review Committee (CTIRC): The Interim Report. II. Examination Relating to Medical Devices*. http://www.mhlw.go.jp (accessed December 2, 2006).

Cohen, Alan B., and Ruth S. Hanf. 2004. *Technology in American Health Care: Policy Directions for Effective Evaluation and Management*. Ann Arbor: The University of Michigan Press.

Colby, Mark A. 2006. "Save our Ailing Health System: Finding an Antidote for the Aging society." *ACCJ Journal* (August): 34–37.

———. 2004. The *Japan Health Care Debate: Diverse Perspectives*, edited by Steve Ziolkowski. Kent, CT: Global Oriental/Folderstone.

Council for Regulatory Reform. 2003. "Third report—Towards the Creation of a Vibrant Japan," (December), http://www.cao.go.jp/kisei/en/pdf.

Curtis, Gerald L. 2002. "Politicians and Bureaucrats: What's Wrong and What's to Be Done." In *Policymaking in Japan: Defining the Role of Politicians.*, edited by Gerald L. Curtis, 1–17, Tokyo: Japan Center for International Exchange.

———. 1999. The *Logic of Japanese Politics: Leaders, Institutions, and the Limits of Change*. New York: Columbia University Press.

Dartmouth Institute for Health Policy and Clinical Practice. *Dartmouth Atlas of Health Care 2008*. Lebanon, NH: The Trustees of Dartmouth College.

Della Porta, Donatella. 2000. "Social Capital, Beliefs in Government, and Political Corruption." In *Disaffected Democracies: What's Troubling the Trilateral Countries?*, edited by Susan J. Pharr and Robert D. Putnam, 202–228, Princeton, NJ: Princeton University Press.

Demske, Gregory E. 2008. U.S. Congress, Senate Special Committee on Aging. *Testimony of Gregory Demske*. Hearing (February 28).

Döhler, Marian. 1997. *Die Regulierung von Professionsgrenzen. Struktur und Entwicklungsdynamik von Gesundheitsberufen im Internationalen Vergleich*. Frankfurt: Campus Verlag.

———. 1992. "Comparing National Patterns of Medical Specialization: A Contribution to the Theory of Professions." *MPIFG Discussion Paper* 92(6).

Dorbeck-Jung, Bärbel R., Diana M. Bowman, and Geert van Calster. 2011. "Governing Nanomedicine: Lessons from Within, and for, the EU Medical Technology Regulatory Framework." Guest Editors' Introduction. *Law and Policy* 33(2): 215–224.

Eaton, Margaret L., and Donald Kennedy. 2007. *Innovation in Medical Technology: Ethical Issues and Challenges*. Baltimore, MD: The Johns Hopkins University.

Edwin O. Reischauer Center for East Asian Studies. *The United States and Japan in 2003: Navigating Uncharted Waters.* Washington, DC: The Paul H. Nitze School of Advanced International Studies, Johns Hopkins University Press.

Emergo Group and Medical Device Summit. 2011. *Medical Device Industry Outlook: A Snapshot of the Medical Device Industry Based on a Survey of Medical Device Professionals.* Austin, TX, 1–15. Available at: www.emergogroup.com.

Eno, Hideo. 2006. "Post-market Obligation in Japan." Paper presented at Japanese Submission Workshop: How to Comply with Japan's Regulatory Requirements (November 8–9). Tokyo, Japan.

Eucomed. 2010. http://www.eucomed.org/Home/portal/whatsnew/10/03/26/japan.aspx.

Eucomed Brussels. 1996. *Eucomed, CEC Meeting—Mutual Recognition Agreements, 15 January 1996.* CORR Nr. 006805.

European Commission. 2013a. *Joint Statement by the President of the European Commission, José Manuel Barroso, the President of the European Council, Herman Van Rompuy, and the Prime Minister of Japan, Shinzo Abe.* Press Release IP/13/276 (2013): http://europa.eu-rapid/press-release_IP-13-276_en.htm (accessed July 20, 2013).

———. 2013b. *A Free Trade Agreement between the EU and Japan.* Memo/137572 sess (June 17, 2013).

———. 2012a. *Proposal for a Regulation of the European Parliament and of the Council on Medical Devices, and Amending Directive 2001/82/EC, Regulation (EC) No. 178/2002 and Regulation (EC) No. 1223/2009.* Brussels (September 26). COM (2012) 542 final—2012/0266 (COD) http://ec.europa.eu/health/medical-devices/documents/revision/index_en.htm?print=true.

———. 2012b. *Proposal for a Regulation of the European Parliament and of the Council on In Vitro Diagnostic Medical* in September 26, 2012. Brussels (September 26). COM(2012) 541 final—2012/0267(COD). Available from http://ec.europa.eu/health/medicaldevices/documents/revision/index_en.htm?print=true.

———. 2008. Directorate-General for Trade. *A Guide to the Mutual Recognition Agreement between the European Community and Japan.*

———. 2005. *Human Tissue-engineered Products: Potential Socio-economic Impacts of a New European Regulatory Framework for Authorization, Supervision, and Vigilance.* A synthesis report prepared by Anne-Katrin Bock and Emilio Rodriguez-Cerezo (JRC-UOTS) and Bärbel Hüsing, Bernhard Bührlen, and Michael Nusser (Fraunhofer Institute for Systems and Innovation Research). Directorate General Joint Research Centre, Technical Report EUR 21838.

Fahy, John, and Fuyuki Taguchi. 1995. "Reassessing the Japanese System." *Sloan Management Review* (Winter): 49–61.

Feder, Barnaby J. "Artificial-joint Makers Settle Kickback Case." *The New York Times,* September 28, 2007, sec. Business Section.

Feldman, Eric A. 2000. *The Ritual of Rights in Japan Law, Society, and Health Policy.* Cambridge: Cambridge University Press.

———. 1999. "HIV and Blood in Japan: Transforming Private Conflict into Public Scandal." In *Blood Feuds: AIDS, Blood, and the Politics of Medical Disaster,* edited by Eric A. Feldman and Ronald Bayer, 59–93. Oxford: Oxford University Press.

———. 1997. "Patients' Rights, Citizens' Movements, and Japanese Legal Cultures." In *Comparing Legal Cultures,* edited by David Nelken, et al.: 215–235. Brookfield, VT: Dartmouth Publishing Company.

———. 1994. "Legal Transplants, Organ Transplants: the Japanese Experience." *Social and Legal Studies* (3): 71–91. London: Sage.

Feldman, Eric A., and Ronald Bayer (eds.). 1999. *AIDS, Blood, and the Politics of Medical Disaster.* Oxford: Oxford University Press.

Finn, Karen. 2010a. "Japan to Speed Up Registration Process for More Devices." *RAJ Devices* (November 28). http://www.rajdevices.com/productsector/medicaldevices/japan-to-speed-up-registration.

———. 2010b."Globalisation Drives Device Regulation." *RAJ Devices* (January 13).

———. 2010c. "Japan Eases Requirements for Certain Class II Devices." *RAJ Devices* (November 9).

Finn, Karen, and Alan Chalmers. "2010 Today." *RAJ Devices.* http://www.rajdevis.com-productsector/medicaldevices/Japan-and-Switzerland-to-exchange.

Foreign Press Center Japan. 2007. *Facts and Figures of Japan.* Tokyo, Japan.

Freddi, George, and James W. Bjorkman. 1989. *Controlling Medical Professionals: The Comparative Politics of Health Governance.* London: Sage.

Freidson, Eliot. 1970a. *Professional Dominance: The Social Structure of Medical Care.* Chicago: Aldine Publishing Company.

———. 1970b. *The Profession of Medicine: A Study of the Sociology of Applied Knowledge.* Chicago: University of Chicago Press.

Fujiwara, Yasuhiro. 1998. "MD Reviewers' Role in the New Anticancer Drug Approval Process in the Newly Established Japanese Regulatory Agency, PMDEC (Pharmaceutical and Medical Devices Evaluation)." *Japanese Journal of Clinical Oncology* 28(11): 653–656.

Fukui, Tsuguya. 2001. "Contribution of Research and Basic and Clinical Science in Japan." *Internal Medicine* 41: 626.

Gary, Allison D., and Yasunori Sone. 1993. *Political Dynamics in Contemporary Japan.* Ithaca: Cornell University Press.

Giroud, Danielle. 2009. "The 2009 Revision of ISO 14155: A True Guidance for Medical Device Companies?" *RAJ Devices* (November 13).

Global Harmonization Task Force (GHTF). 2009. 12th Annual Conference Proceedings. *Final Documents: Guidance on How to Handle Information Concerning Vigilance Reporting Related to Medical Devices* (May 12–14). Toronto, Canada.

———. 2007a. 11th Annual Conference Proceedings. Washington, DC. October 3–4.

———. 2007b. *Clinical Evidence—Key Definitions and Concepts, Study Group 5.* SG5/N1R8: 2007.

———. 2006a. *Final Documents. Medical devices post market surveillance: global guidance for adverse event reporting for medical devices.* GHTF/SG2/N54R8.

———. 2006b. *Final Documents: Guidance on How to Handle Information Concerning Vigilance Reporting Related to Medical Devices.*

———. 2006c. 10th Annual Conference Proceedings. Conference design for patient safety in a global regulatory model. Lübeck, Germany. June 28–30.

Goodman, Clifford. 2000. Keynote Lecture. Paper presented at the International Society of Technology Assessment in Health Care (ISTAHC), The Hague, The Netherlands. June 21.

———. 2002. The *Value of Diagnostics, Innovation, Adoption, and Diffusion into Health Care*. Lewin Group, Inc.

Gross, Ames. 2005. "Japan's New Regulatory Environment for Medical Devices." *Pacific Bridge Medical* (June). www.pacificbridgemedical.com.

———. 1997. "Keeping Up with Changes in the Japanese Medical Market." *Medical Device & Diagnostic Industry* (May). http://www.devicelink.com/mddi/archive/97/05/019.html.

Gross, Ames, and Caroline Tran. 2002. "Device Regulation in Asia: An Update." *Medical Device Link*. http://www.devicelink.com/mddi/archive/0210/003.html, 1–5.

Gross, Ames, and John Minot. 2009. "Japan Quality Audits 2009." *Pacific Bridge Medical* (January), http://www.pacificbridgemedical.com/publications/japan/Kapn_Quality_Audits2009/htm.

Gross, Ames, and Momoko Hirose. 2009. "Updates on the Medical Device Markets in Japan, China and India." *Pacific Bridge Medical*. http://www.pacificbridge-medical.com/publications/asia2009_updates_on_medical devices (accessed August 1, 2011).

———. 2007. "Medical Device Reimbursement in Japan." *Pacific Bridge Medical* (January). www.pacificbridgemedical.com.

Gross, Ames, and Nancy Loh. 2006. "Medical Device Regulatory Update: China and Japan." *Medical Device & Diagnostic Industry* (September/October). http://www.pacificbridgemedical.com/publications/html/Medical_Device_Regulatory_Update.

Gusmano, Michael K., Victor G. Rodwin, and D. Weisz. 2010. *Health Care in World Cities: New York, London and Paris*. Baltimore, Maryland: Johns Hopkins University Press.

Hall, Peter. 2003. "Aligning Ontology and Methodology in Comparative Research." In *Comparative Historical Analysis in the Social Sciences*, edited by James Mahoney and Dietrich Rueschemeyer, 373–404. Cambridge: Cambridge University Press.

Hancher, Leigh, and Michael Moran. 1989. "Organizing Regulatory Space." In *Capitalism, Culture and Regulation*, 271–299. Oxford: Clarendon Press.

Hartcher, Peter. 1998. *The Ministry: How Japan's Most Powerful Institute Endangers World Markets*. Boston: Harvard Business School Press.

Hasegawa, Tomonori. "New Development of Health Sector Reform in Japan" (Power Point Presentation, n.d., courtesy author, technical advisor at the Council for the Promotion of Regulatory Reform, Cabinet Office.)

———. 2002. "Quality Improvement in Health Care; an example of Japan." Presentation, no location, courtesy author.

Hasegawa, Toshihiko. 2007. "New Challenges for Patient Safety." Paper presented at the International Symposium on Health Policy and Management, May 27, Tokyo, Japan.

———. 2002. "Research Strategy and Activity on Patient Safety in Japan." Tokyo: National Institute of Public Health.

Hayao, Kenji. 1993. *The Japanese Prime Minister and Public Policy*. Pittsburgh, PA: University of Pittsburgh Press.

Heady, Ferrel. 2001. *Public Administration: A Comparative Perspective* (5th ed.), New York: Marcel Drekker.

Higuchi, Norio. 2007a. *Thinking about Medicine and Law* [Iryou to Ho wo kangaeru]. Tokyo: Yuhikaku Publishing.

———. 2007b. *Bioethics and the Law* [Seimei Rinri to Ho], vols. 1 and 2. Nagoya City, Japan: Kobundo.

———. 2007c. "Self-regulation and Excessive Reaction to Personal Health Information Protection in Japan." *University of Tokyo Journal of Law and Politics* 4 (Spring 2007c): 108–109.

———. 2007d. "Personal information and excessive reaction to personal health information protection in Japan." *University of Tokyo Journal of Law and Politics* 4 (Spring 2007d): 99–107.

———. 2005. "Medical Information and Privacy in the Information Society." *University of Tokyo Journal of Law and Politics* 2 (Spring): 73–81.

Hirao, Tomohiro. 2007. "Hospital Strategic Management in Japan Focusing on University Hospitals." Paper presented at the International Symposium on Health Policy and Management, May 27, Tokyo, Japan.

Hirayama, Kiyomi, Naohisa Fukuda, Hitoshi Satoh, Katsumi Itoh, Kiyoshi Chiba, Yutaka Nakae, Masayuki Takezawa, Kuniko Gotoh, and Naoto Uemura. 2005a. "Checklist for GCP Compliance Investigation (Medical Institution)." *Quality Assurance Journal* 9: 120–139.

———. 2005b. "Overseas GCP Inspections by the Japanese Regulatory Agency: A Systematic Review of 13 cases (1998–2003)." *Quality Assurance Journal* 9: 14–21.

Hirose, Makoto. 2006a. "Applications for Biological Products." Paper presented at Japan Submission Workshop, November 8–9, Tokyo, Japan.

———. 2006b. "Notices Concerning In-vitro Diagnostics." Paper presented at Japan Submission Workshop, November 8–9, Tokyo, Japan.

Hodges, Christopher. 2011. "The Regulation of Medicines and Medical Device." In Andrew Grubb, Judith Laing, Jean McHale, and Ian Kennedy (eds.), ch.17, *Principles of Medical Law*. Oxford: Oxford University Press.

———. 2005. *European Regulation of Consumer Product Safety*. Oxford: Oxford University Press.

Hollingsworth, J. Rogers. 1997. "How and Why Do SSPs Change? The Cases of Japan, Germany and the USA." In *Contemporary Capitalism: The Embeddednes of Institutions*, edited by J. Rogers Hollingsworth and Robert Boyer, 265–310. Cambridge: Cambridge University Press.

Horiguchi, Hikaru. 2007. "Challenges to Patient Access and Potential Market and Regulatory Solutions." Paper presented at a Leadership Dialogue for Stakeholders and Policy Leaders from Japan and the United States, April 21–23, Karuizawa, Japan.

Ikegami, Naoki. 2009. "Containing Healthcare Expenditures in Japan." Lecture, November 25, Mailman School of Public Health, Columbia University.

———. 2008. "Japan, Health System of." In *International Encyclopedia of Public Health* 1(4), Kris Heggenhougen and Stella Quah (eds.), 1–8. San Diego: Academic Press.

———. 2007. "Overview of the Japanese Health System." April 21–23 at a Leadership Dialogue for Stakeholders and Policy Leaders from Japan and the United States, Karuizawa, Japan.

———. 2004. "Japan's Health Care System: Containing Costs and Attempting Reform." *Health Affairs* (May–June): 26–36.

Ikegami, Naoki, and John Creighton Campbell. 2008. "Dealing with the Medical Axis-of-Power: The Case of Japan." *Health Economics, Policy and Law* 3(2): 107–113.

———. 1999. "Health Care Reform in Japan: The Virtues of Muddling Through." *Health Affairs* 18(3): 56–75.

Ikegami, Naoki, Byung-Kwang Yoo, Hideki Hashimoto, Masatoshi Matsumoto, Hiraya Ogata, Akira Babazono, Ryo Watanabe, Kenji Shibuya, Bong-Min Jang, Michael R. Reich. 2011. "Japanese Universal Health Coverage: Evolution, Achievements, and Challenges." *The Lancet* 378 (September): 1106–1115. www. thelancet.com.

Institute of Health Policy. 2007. *Public Surveys.* Tokyo: University of Tokyo, http:// www.healthpolicy-institute.org/research/PublicOpinionSurvey2007.pdf.

———. 2006a. *Public Surveys.* University of Tokyo, http://healthpolicy-institute. or/eng/research/PublicOpinionSurvey2006.pdf.

———. 2006b. *Healthcare Reform: Unfinished Agenda—Issues and Choices as Defined by the Japanese Public.* University of Tokyo.

Institute of Medicine. 2011a. *Medical Devices and the Public's Health. The FDA 510(k) Clearance Process at 35 Years.* Washington, DC: The National Academies Press.

———. 2011b. *Public Health Effectiveness of the FDA 510(k) Clearance Process: Measuring Post-Market Performance and Other Select Topics.* (Workshop report.) Washington, DC: The National Academies Press.

———. 2001. *Responsible Research: A Systems Approach to Protecting Research Participants.* Washington, DC: The National Academies Press.

Ishikawa, Hiroshi. 2009a. "Adverse event reporting—the traceability of concerned devices and reporting of events." Paper presented May 12–14, GHTF 12th Annual Conference Proceedings. Toronto, Canada.

———. 2009b. "Realizing the Value of Technology." Paper presented May 12–14, GHTF 12th Annual Conference Proceedings. Toronto, Canada.

Japan Federation of Medical Devices Association (JFMDA). *Pharmaceutical Affairs Law—New Regulations Effective in 2005.* Yakinji Nippo, Ltd.

Japan Federation of Medical Devices Association (JFMDA), 2007. *Outline of the Japan Federation of Medical Devices Associations.* Tokyo, Japan. http://www. jfmda.gr.jp/e/index.html.

———. 2006. "Trends of Medical Devices Regulation in Japan, the US and Europe and Developing Markets." The 24th International Medical Devices Seminar, Tokyo, Japan. December 11.

Japan Public Health Association. 2007. *Public Health in Japan 2007.* Tokyo.

Japan Times. 2008. "Basic Accord Ends Hepatitis C Legal Fights" (January 16): 2.

Kadonaga, Sonosuke, Ludwig Kanzler, and Yukako Yokoyama. 2008. "Addressing Japan's Health Care Cost Challenge." *The McKinsey Quarterly* (May): 1–11.

Kakizoe, Tadao. 2008. "Japan Must Improve Clinical Trial Infrastructure." *The Daily Yomiuri* (January 20), sec. Commentary.

Kasahara, Hidehiko. 1999. *Nihon no iryougyousei sono rekishi to kadai* [Japan's Medical Administration: Its History and Challenges]. Tokyo: Kei University Press.

Katzenstein, Peter. 2000. "Confidence, Trust, International Relations." In *Disaffected Democracies: What's Troubling the Trilateral Countries?* Edited by Susan J. Pharr and Robert D. Putnam, 121–148, Princeton, NJ: Princeton University Press.

Kawabuchi, Koichi. 2006. "Socio-economics on Care for the Elderly Patients with Hip Fracture." *Nippon Rinsho* 64(9) (September): 1589–1596.

Kawabuchi, Koichi, and Keiko Kajitani. 2007a. "The Fifth Revision and the Beyond—Health Care Reform in Japan." *Japan Hospitals* 25 (January): 11–18.
———. 2007b. "Issues in Expansion of DPC." *Japan Hospitals* 26 (December): 19–30.
Kawabuchi, Koichi, and Shigeru Sugihara. 2006. "The Volume-outcome Relationship in Japan. The Case of Percutaneous Transluminal Coronary Angioplasty (PTCA). Volume on Mortality of Acute Myocardial Infarction (AMI) Patients." In *Health Care Issues in the US and Japan*, edited by David A. Wise and Naohiro Yashiro, 113–140. Chicago: University of Chicago Press.
Kelemen, R. Daniel. 2011. *Eurolegalism: The Transformation of Law and Politics in the European Union*. Cambridge, MA: Harvard University Press.
Kenny, Maureen. 2010a. "Approval for Revised International Medical Device GCP Standard." *RAJ Devices* (November 11).
———. 2010b. Editorial. *Regulatory Affairs* (September/October). www.regulatoryaffairs.medtech.com.
Kerbo, Harold R., and John A. McKinstry. 1995. *Who Rules Japan? The Inner Circles of Economic and Political Power*. New York: Praeger.
Kessler, Larry G. 2007a. "The Global Harmonization Task Force, Clinical Evidence—Key Definitions and Concepts, Study Group 5." SG5/N1R8: 2007.
———. 2007b. "Introduction to the Action Plan for 2007–2010: Path Forward for the Global Harmonization Task Force."
Kimura, Saburo. 2007. "US Medical Device Industry in Japan—Its Past, Present, and Future." Paper presented at ACCJ MD&D Subcommittee, December 11, US Embassy, Japan.
Kleinknecht, Alfred, Kees van Montfort, and Erik Brouwer. 2002. "The Non-trivial Choice between Innovation Indicators." *Economics of Innovation and New Technology* 11(2): 109–121.
Kondo, James M. 2007. "Survey Results of the Status Quo in Japan—Patient Opinion and Health Policy." Paper presented April 21–23, Leadership Dialogues for Stakeholders and Policy Leaders from Japan and the United States, Karuizawa, Japan.
———. 2006. "Healthcare Reform: Unfinished Agenda Issues and Choices as Defined by the Japanese Public." September 8. Available at http://www.healthpolicy-institute.org/eng/research/PublicOpinionSurvey2006.
———. 2006. "Japanese Public's Perceptions of Healthcare Policy Priorities." Available at http://www.healthpolicy-institute.org/eng/research/PublicOpinionSurvey2006-PdF.
———. 2006. "Survey of Cancer Patients and Their Families." March 19. Available at http://www.healthpolicy-institute.org/eng/research/cancerpatientsandtheirfamilies.
———. 2005. "The Iron Triangle of Japan's Healthcare." *British Medical Journal* 330(7482): 55–56.
Kondo, Tatsuya. "Message from the Chief Executive, PMDA." Available at http://wwww.pmda.jp/English/about/message (accessed September 17, 2010, and January 9, 2014).
Kudo, Hiroko, and Jeroen Maesschalck. 2005. "Japan's National Public Service Ethics Law: Background, Contents, and Impact." Paper presented at Ethics and Integrity of Governance: The First Transatlantic Dialogue, June 2–5, Leuven, Belgium.

Kuroyanagi, Tatsuo. 2005. *Medical Facilities and Administrative Justice Decisions* [Iryô shisetsu to shiho handan]. 5th printing, Hanrei times Sha (Judicial Times Company).

———. 2002. *Medical Incidents and Judicial Judgment* [Iryoijiko to shihou handan]. Tokyo: Taimuzu-sha.

Kuroyanagi, Tatsuo, Kozo Takase, and Junji Maeda. 2005. *The Prescription of Medical Lawsuits from A to Z.* Tokyo: Hanrei Times Co. Ltd.

———. 2004. *Wakariyasui Iryousaibansho Housen* [Easy to Understand Medical Lawsuits]. Tokyo: Hanrei Taimusuä.

Leflar, Robert B. 2009. "Unnatural deaths, criminal sanctions, and medical quality improvement in Japan." *Yale Journal of Health Policy, Law and Ethics* IX (1): 101–136.

———. 1996. "Informed Consent and Patients' Rights in Japan." *Houston Law Review* 33(1) (Spring): 1–112.

Leflar, Robert B., and Futoshi Iwata. 2006. "Regulating for Patient Safety: The Law's Response to Medical Errors; Medical Error as Reportable Event, as Tort, as Crime: A Transpacific Comparison." *Zeitschrift für Japanisches Recht/Journal of Japanese law*: 39–76.

———. 2005. "Regulating for Patient Safety: The Law's Response to Medical Errors; Medical Error as Reportable Event, as Tort, as Crime: A Transpacific Comparison." *Widener Law Review* 12: 1–38.

L. E. K. Acumen Japan, LLC. 2005. *ACCJ Toolbox Analysis, Final Results*: 1–40.

Leichter, Howard M. 1979. *A Comparative Approach to Policy Analysis.* Cambridge: Cambridge University Press.

Lévi-Faur, David. 2005. "The Political Economy of Legal Globalization: Juridification, Adversarial Legalism, and Responsive Regulation: A Comment." *International Organization*: 451–426.

Lewin Group, Inc. 2002. *Outlook for Medical Technology Innovation.* Prepared for AdvaMed.

Lipset, Seymour Martin. 1996. *American Exceptionalism: A Double-edged Sword.* New York: W.W. Norton & Company.

Lowi, Theodore J. 1973. "What Political Scientists Don't Need to Ask about Policy Analysis." *Policy Studies Journal* 2(1): 61–67.

———. 1972. "Four Systems of Policy, Politics, and Choice." *Public Administration Review (PAR)* 32(4) (July–August): 298–310.

Ludwig, Edwards J., chairman, president, and chief executive officer, Becton, Dickinson and Company, and chairman of the board of AdvaMed. 2006. "Before the International Trade Commission on Medical Devices and Equipment: Competitive Conditions Affecting US Trade in Japan and Other Principal Foreign Markets," Investigation Number 332–474 Cong., July 11 session.

Marmor, Theodore R., Richard Freeman, and Kieke Okma. 2005. "Comparative Perspectives and Policy Learning in the World of Health Care." *Journal of Comparative Policy Analysis* 7(4): 331–348.

Marmor, Theodore R., Kieke Okma and Richard Freeman. 2009. *Comparative Studies and the Politics of Modern Medical Care.* New Haven, CT: Yale University Press.

Marmor, Theodore R., and Claus Wendt. 2011. "Conceptual Framework for Comparative Healthcare Politics and Policy." Paper presented at the

European Health Policy Group meeting, September 22–23, London School of Economics.

Matsumoto, Kazuhiko, Yoshihiro Arakawa, Ryuji Koike, Tetsuya Nakamura, Hideki Hanaoka, Masato Honma, Hirohisa Yoshizawa. 2013. "Centralization of Reviews by IRBs in University Hospitals: Consideration of Collaborative IRB in University Hospital Clinical Trial Alliance. *Rinsho yajuri/Japanese Journal of Pharmacology and Therapeutics* 44(3): 207–215.

Matsumura, Kazuya. 2006. "Preclinical Testing Requirements—Stability Testing Requirements." Paper presented at AdvaMed, Submission Workshop, November 8–9, Tokyo, Japan.

Matsutani, Yukio. 2007. "MTLF Forum Report: A Special Program." Paper presented at a Policy Leadership Dialogue for Stakeholders and Policy Leaders from Japan and the United States, April 21–23, Karuizawa, Japan.

Maxwell, Amanda. 2012. "EU Medtech Groups Optimistic Over Commission's FTA Plan with Japan." http://www.rajpharma.com (received August 8. 2012).

McCall Rosenbluth, Frances, and Michael F. Thies. 2010. *Japan Transformed: Political Change and Economic Restructuring.* Princeton, NJ: Princeton University Press.

Meier, Barry. 2009. *New York Times.* "Costs Surge for Medical Devices, but Benefits Are Opaque" (November 5).

Minami, Kazutomo. 2004. *Konna iryoude iidesuka—nihonde okonawareteiru iryou, doitsude okonawareteiru iryou* [Is this Medical Care Good Enough? Medical Care in Japan and Germany]. Tokyo: Haru Shobo.

Ministry of Education, Culture, Sports, Science, and Technology. 2006. "Reform of Japan's Science and Technology System." In *White Paper on Science and Technology,* http://www.mext.jp./english (accessed January 19, 2008).

Ministry of Foreign Affairs (MOFA). 2007. "Sixth Report to the Leaders on the US-Japan Regulatory Reform and Competition Policy Initiative." June 6.

Ministry of Health, Labour, and Welfare (MHLW). 2007. Clinical Trial Issue Review Committee (CTIRC). http://www.go.jp/english/index.html.

———. *Section II: Examination Relating to Medical Devices.*

———. *Section III: Examination Relating to Advanced Medical Technology in Life Science.*

———. *Ministerial Ordinance: Good Clinical Practice for Medical Devices.* Public Law MHLW Ordinance No. 36. 2005.

———. *On Clinical Trials of Medical Devices Conducted Overseas.* FS/Notification No. 0331006.

Ministry of Health and Welfare (MHW). *On Data from Clinical Trials of Medical Devices Conducted Overseas.* MHW/PAB Notification No 476.

Mitsumori, Yoshio. 2009a. "New Japanese Prime Minister Vows Changes to Healthcare." *Medical Product Outsourcing Magazine* (November/December). All available at http://www.mpo-mag.com.

———. 2009b. "News from Japan. Still Coping with Japan's 'Device Lag.'" *Medical Product Outsourcing Magazine* (July/August).

———. 2009c. "Japan's PMDA Kicks off Improvement Program." *Medical Product Outsourcing Magazine* (May).

———. 2009d. "Japan Is Continuing Efforts to Speed Up Device Reviews." *Medical Product Outsourcing Magazine* (January/February).

———— 2008. "Becoming a Global Player: Japan Moves to Boost Its Medical Technology Infrastructure." *Medical Product Outsourcing Magazine* (December).

————. 2007a. "The Latest Regulatory Environment for Medical Devices in Japan." *Medical Product Outsourcing Magazine* (January).

————. 2007b. "New Report Exemplifies Japan's Slow Approval Process." *Medical Product Outsourcing Magazine* (May).

————. 2006a. "Japan's Political Shakeup: A New Cabinet Brings New Policy." *Medical Product Outsourcing Magazine* (November/December): 34–35.

————. 2006b. "Charting Important Change in Japan's Device Review Regulations." *Medical Product Outsourcing Magazine* (October): 26–28.

Miyamoto, Masao. 1994. *Straitjacket Society: An Insider's Irreverent View of Bureaucratic Japan*. Tokyo: Kodansha International.

Mladovsky, Philipa, Sherry Merkur, Elias Mossialos, and Martin McKee. 2009. "Lifelong Learning and Physician Revalidation in Europe." *Euro Observer: The Health Policy Bulletin of the European Observatory on Health Systems and Policies* 11(2) (Summer): 1–12.

MTLF forum report, special program. 2007. A Leadership Dialogue for Stakeholders and Policy Leaders from Japan and the United States, April 21–23, Karuizawa, Japan. Report written by Susan Bartlett Foote, School of Public Health. University of Minnesota, Minneapolis.

MTLF Forum report. 2005. "Tapping Medical Technology to Improve Quality and Efficiency in Health Care: An International Dialogue." A Leadership Conference for Stakeholders and Policy Leaders from Japan and the United States, May 2–5, Washington, DC.

MTLF. 2001. *Risk and Rewards in Medical Technology Innovation: Conflict of Interest at the Academic/Industry Surface*, edited by Susan Bartlett Foot, 1–10. Palo Alto, CA: Stanford University Press.

Muramatsu, Michio, and Ellis S. Krauss. 1996. "Japan: The Paradox of Success." In *Lessons from Experience: Experiential Learning in Eight Democracies*, edited by Johan P. Olsen and B. Guy Peters, 214–242. Oslo: Scandinavian University Press.

Muraoka, Akira. 2005. "Renovation of Postgraduate Clinical Training System for MDs in Japan." MHLW, PDF presentation dated January 24, Tokyo, Japan.

Naito, Masaaki. 2006. "Global Harmonization Task Force Working Towards Global Harmonization in Medical Device Regulation." Conference proceedings. Paper presented at the 10th Global Harmonization Task Force (GHTF) Conference Design for Patient Safety in a Global Regulatory Model, June 29, Lübeck, Germany.

Nakajima, K., Y. Kurata, and H. Takeda. 2005. "A Web-based Incident Reporting System and Multidisciplinary Collaborative Projects for Patient Safety in a Japanese Hospital." *Quality and Safety in Health Care* 14, http://qshc.bmj.com/cgi/content/abstract/14/2/123.

Nakajima, Kazue, Catherine Keyes, Tatsuo Kurayanagi, and Kozo Tatara. 2001. "Medical Malpractice and Legal Resolutions Systems in Japan." *JAMA* 285(12): 1632–1640.

Nakamura, Robert T. 1990. "The Japan External Trade Organization and Import Promotion: A Case Study in the Implementation of Symbolic Goals." In *Implementation and Public Policy: Opening Up the Black Box*, edited by Donald J. Calista and Dennis J. Palumbo, 67–86. New York: Greenwood Press.

Nakatoni, Yukiko. 2006. "Direction of Reimbursement for Medical Devices in Japan." Paper presented, AdvaMed Annual Meeting, October 30, 2006 (PDF, courtesy Dr. Nakatoni).

Nakayama, Shigeru. 2001. "The International Exchange of Scientific Information." In *The Social History of Science and Technology in Contemporary Japan: The Occupation Period 1945–1952*, edited by Shigeru Nakayama, Junio Gotō, and Hitoshi Yoshioka. Vol. 1, 249–260. Melbourne: Trans Pacific Press.

Nakayama, Shigeru, Junio Gotō, and Hitoshi Yoshioka (eds.). 2006. *A Social History of Science and Technology in Contemporary Japan: High Economic Growth Period 1960–1969.* Vol. 3. Melbourne: Trans Pacific Press.

———. 2005a. *A Social History of Science and Technology in Contemporary Japan: Road to Self-Reliance 1952.* Vol. 2. Melbourne: Trans Pacific Press.

———. 2005b. *A Social History of Science and Technology in Contemporary Japan: The Occupation Period 1945–1952.* Vol. 1. Melbourne: Trans Pacific Press.

National Policy Unit (NPU). 2012. *Rebirth of Japan: A Comprehensive Strategy Cabinet Decision,* July 31.

NHK TV (Japan Broadcasting Corporation). 2006. "Why Is It Expensive? The Price of Medical Devices—Unknown Price Disparity." December 9 TV program on DVD (translated from the Japanese by Chiomi Kasahara, former graduate student at the City University of New York's Graduate Center).

Nomi, Yoshihisa. 1999. "Medical Liability in Japanese Law." In *Modern Trends in Tort Law,* edited by E. Hondius, 27–39. Kluwer Law International.

Nottage, Luke. 2005. "Comparing Product Safety and Liability Law in Japan from Minamata to Mad Cows—and Mitsubishi." In *Product Liability in Comparative Perspective,* edited by Duncan Fairgrieve, 334–340. Cambridge: Cambridge University Press.

———. 2004. *Product Safety and Liability Law in Japan: From Minamata to Mad Cows.* London: Routledge Curzon, Taylor & Francis Group.

Organization for Economic Cooperation and Development. 2011a. *Help Wanted? Providing and Paying for Long-Term Care.* Paris: OECD.

———. 2011b. *OECD Health Data 2011: How Does Japan Compare?* Paris: OECD. Available from http://www.oecd.org/longtermcare (accessed July 5, 2011).

———. 2010. *Health at a Glance: Europe 2010.* Paris: OECD.

Ohki, Takao. 2007. "Advanced Medical Devices Save Lives: Vascular Surgery." Paper presented at a Leadership Dialogue for Stakeholders and Policy Leaders from Japan and the United States, April 21–23, Karuizawa, Japan.

Oliver, Adam. 2003. "Health Economic Evaluation in Japan: A Case of One Aspect of Health Technology Assessment." *Health Policy* 63: 97–104.

Oliver, Adam, Elias Mossialos, and Ray Robinson. 2004. "Health Technology Assessment and Its Influence on Health-care Priority Setting." *International Journal of Technology Assessment in Health Care* 20(1): 1–10.

Ono, Shunsuke, Yasuo Kodama, Taku Nagao, and Satoshi Toyoshima. 2002. "The Quality of Conduct in Japanese Clinical Trials: Deficiencies Found in GCP Inspections." *Controlled Clinical Trials* 23: 29–41.

Otake, Hideo. 2000. "Political Mistrust and Party Dealignment in Japan." In *Disaffected Democracies: What's Troubling the Trilateral Countries?,* edited by Susan J. Pharr and Robert D. Putnam, 291–310. Princeton, NJ: Princeton University Press.

Pammolli, Fabio, Massimo Riccaboni, Claudia Oglialoro, Laura Magazzini, Gianluca Baio, and Nicola Salerno. 2005. *Medical Devices: Competitiveness and Impact on Health Expenditure.* Rome: CERM (Competitiveness, Markets and Regulation).

Pempel, T. J. 1992. "Japan's Creative Conservativism: Continuity under Challenge." In *The Comparative History of Public Policy* (2nd ed.), edited by Francis G. Castles, 149–191. Cambridge: Polity Press.

Pempel, T. J., and Michio Muramatsu. 1995. "The Japanese Bureaucracy and Economic Development: Structuring a Proactive Civil Service." In *The Japanese Bureaucracy and Economic Development: Catalyst of Change,* edited by Hyung-Ki Kim, Michio Muramatsu, and T. J. Pempel, 19–76. Oxford: Clarendon Press.

Pharma Japan. 2006. "Study Group on 'Device Lag' Holds 1st Meeting."

Pharmaceutical Affairs Law, Enforcement Ordinance, Enforcement Regulations & Law for the Pharmaceuticals and Medical Devices Agency 2005–2006. Yakuji Nippo, Ltd.

Pharmaceutical Affairs Study Group, ed. 2005–2007. *The Pharmaceutical Affairs Law, Enforcement Ordinance and Enforcement Regulations 2005/07.* Yakuji Nippo, Ltd.

Pharmaceuticals and Medical Devices Agency (PMDA). *Roadmap for the PMDA International Visions—April 2013.* All sources available from http://www.pmda.go.jp and http://www.pmda.jp/index-e.html.

——. "Profile of Services, Fiscal Year 2010."

——. "Profile of Services, Fiscal Year 2010: Summary of Relief Services for Adverse Health Effects."

——. "Fiscal Year Annual Report, 2009."

——. "Profile of Services, Fiscal Year 2008."

——. "Quality Management System Inspection of Medical Devices in Japan." 2007.

——. "Basic Ideas for Multi-national Clinical Trials." April 2006.

——. "Our Mission: Relief, Review, Safety." April 2006.

——. "Profile of File of Services, 2006."

——. "Annual Report, Fiscal Year 2005."

——. "Medical safety information, 2004" PFSB, MHLW, 253.

Pharr, Susan J. 2000. "Officials' Misconduct and Public Distrust: Japan and the Tri-lateral Democracies." In *Disaffected Democracies. What's Troubling the Trilateral Countries?,* edited by Susan J. Pharr and Robert D. Putnam, 173–201. Princeton, NJ: Princeton University Press.

Pierson, Paul, and Theda Skocpol. 2002. "Historical Institutionalism in Contemporary Political Science." In *Political Science: The State of the Discipline,* edited by Ira Katznelson and Helen V. Millner, 693–721. New York: W. W. Norton.

Prime Minister of Japan and His Cabinet. 2007. "'Innovation 25': Creating the Future, Challenging Unlimited Possibilities." Interim report, executive summary by the Innovation 25 strategy council.

Richardson, Bradley. 1997. *Japanese Democracy: Power, Coordination, and Performance.* New Haven, CT: Yale University Press.

Rodwin, Marc A. 2011a. *Conflicts of Interest and the Future of Medicine: The United States, France and Japan.* New York: Oxford University Press.

——. 2011b. "Coping with physicians' conflicts of interest in Japan." In *Conflicts of Interest and the Future of Medicine: The United States, France and Japan,* 184–203. Oxford: Oxford University Press.

———. 2011c. "Reforming Pharmaceutical Industry-Physician Financial Relationships: Lessons from the United States, France, and Japan," *Journal of Law, Medicine & Ethics* (Winter): 662–670.

———. 2012. "Conflicts of Interest, Institutional Corruption, and Pharma: An Agenda for Reform." *Legal Studies Research Paper Series: Research Paper 12–40*, October 16. Available at http://ssm.com/abstract=2162597. Also published in *Journal of Law, Medicine & Ethics* (Fall 2012), 511–522.

———. 1993. *Medicine, Money and Morals: Physicians' Conflicts of Interest.* New York: Oxford University Press.

Rodwin, Marc A., and Atoz Etsuji Okamoto. 2000. "Physicians' Conflict of Interests in Japan and the United States: Lessons for the United States." *Journal of Health Politics, Policy and Law* 25(2) (April): 343–375.

Rodwin, Victor G., and Michael K. Gusmano. 2006. *Growing Older in World Cities: New York, London, Paris and Tokyo.* Nashville, TN: Vanderbilt University Press.

Rosenthal, Elizabeth. 2013. "The growing popularity of having surgery overseas." *The New York Times* (August 6). http://www.nytimes.com (accessed August 7, 2013).

Sakamoto, Noriko, Shoichi Maeda, Noraki Ikeda, Hiromi Ishibashi, and Koichi Nobutomo. 2002. "The Use of Medical Experts in Medical Malpractice Litigation in Japan." *Medicine, Science, and the Law* 42(3): 201.

Schaede, Ulrike. 2008. *Choose and Focus: Japanese Business Strategies for the 21st Century.* Ithaca, NY: Cornell University Press.

Schlesinger, Mark (ed.). 2005. "Legacies and Latitude in European Health Policy." Special issue. *Journal of Health Politics, Policy and Law* 30 (1–2) (February–April).

Schwartz, Frank J. 1998. *Advice and Consent: The Politics of Consultation in Japan.* Cambridge: Cambridge University Press.

Schwartz, Frank J., and Susan J. Pharr (eds.). 2003. *The State of Civil Society in Japan.* Cambridge: Cambridge University Press.

"Science Policy: Japan Picks up the 'Innovation' Mantra." 2007. *Science.* April 13, 186.

Sharma, Vibha. 2010. "UK MHRA and Japan's PMDA Agree on Sharing Confidential Data on Therapeutic Products." *RAJ Devices*, http://www.rajdevices.com/productsector/medicaldevices/UK-MHRA-and-Japan-PMDA. (See also "UK MHRA and Japan PMDA Agree on Sharing Confidential Data on Therapeutic Products," www.regulatoryaffairsmedtech.com, November/December: 41.)

Shibato, Masako. 2005. *Japan and Germany Under the US Occupation: A Comparative Analysis of Post-War Education Reform.* Lanham: Lexington Books.

Shibuja, Kenji, Hideki Hashimoto, Naoki Ikegami, Akihiro Neshi, Tetsuya Tanimoto, Hiroaki Miyata, Keizo Takemi, and Michael R. Reich. 2011. "Future of Japan's System of Good Health at Low Cost with Equity: Beyond Universal Coverage." *The Lancet* 378 (9798): 1265–1273. October 1 [doi: 10.1016/S0140-6736(11)61098-2].

Shiraishi, Junichi. 2007. "MTLF Forum Report: A Leadership Dialogue for Stakeholders and Policy Leaders from Japan and the United States." April 21–23, Karuizawa, Japan.

Stark, Nancy J. 2011. "Key Revisions to Medical Device Clinical Investigations Standard ISO 14155." *RAJ Devices*, http://www.rajdevices.com.

Starr, Paul. 1982. *The Social Transformation of American Medicine: The Rise of a Sovereign Profession and the Making of a Vast Industry.* New York: Basic Books, Inc.

Steinbrook, Robert. 2009. "Controlling Conflicts of Interest—Proposals from the Institute of Medicine." *New England Journal of Medicine* 360, http://www.nejm.org-doi/full/10.1056(NEJMp0810200 (accessed January 11, 2011).

Steslicke, William A. 1973. *Doctors in Politics: The Political Life of the Japan Medical Association.* New York: Praeger Publishers.

Stettler, Christoph, Simon Wandel, Sabin Allemann et al. 2007. "Outcomes Associated with Drug-eluting and Bare-metal Stents: A Collaborative Network Meta-analysis." *The Lancet* 370(9591): 937–948.

Stevens, Rosemary. 2006. "Medical Specialization as American Health Policy: Interweaving Public and Private Roles." In *History and Health Policy in the United States: Putting the Past Back In,* edited by Rosemary A. Stevens, Charles E. Rosenberg, and Lawton R. Burns, 44–81. New Brunswick, NJ: Transaction Publishers.

———. 2003. *Medical Practice in Modern England: The Impact of Specialization and State Medicine.* New Brunswick, NJ: Transaction Publishers.

Stone, Deborah A. 2002. *Policy Paradox: The Art of Political Decision Making* (revised edition). New York: W. W. Norton & Company.

Süddeutsche Zeitung, June 26, 2013.

Suleiman, Ezra. 2003. *Dismantling Democratic States.* Princeton, NJ: Princeton University Press.

Swiontkowski, Marc. 2007. "Regulatory shortcomings and potential solutions: provider community responsibility: The example of BMP-2 (bone)." Paper presented at a Policy Leadership Dialogue for Stakeholders and Policy Leaders from Japan and the United States, 21–23 April 2007, Karuizawa, Japan.

Synovate Health Care. 2007. "The Japanese Market in Transition—Time for Western Multinationals to Up the Ante?" Presentation at PBIRG 2007, Education Workshop, September 27–29, Tokyo, Japan.

Tadashi, Yamamoto. 1999. *Deciding the Public Good: Governance and Civil Society in Japan.* Tokyo: Japan Center for International Change.

Takae, Shinichi. 2007. "Japanese Quality Systems Auditing—Current and Future." Paper presented at 11th Conference of the Global Harmonization Task Force, October 3–4, Washington, DC.

Takakura, Nobuyuki. 2003. "Discussion on Insurance Reimbursement for Medical Devices and Vision of Medical Device Industry in Japan." Economic Affairs Division, Health Policy Bureau, MHLW, PDF presentation dated September 9.

Talcott, Paul. 1999. "Japan's Next Big Bang: Healthcare Reform Implications for US Policy." Paper presented at Session III: Healthcare Reform and Global Trade, Washington, DC, February 17.

Tan, Tina. 2013a. "Japan Gives Go-ahead to Medtech-specific Regulatory System." December 11. http://www.rajpharma.com.

———. 2013b. "Japan to Build up Regulatory Muscle." May 31, http://www.rajpharma.com.

Tanabe, Kuniaki. 1997. "Social Policy in Japan: Building a Welfare State in a Conservative One Dominant Party System." In *State and Administration in Japan and Germany: A Comparative Perspective on Continuity and Change,* edited by Michio Muramatsu and Frieder Naschold, 107–156. Berlin: Walter de Gruyter.

Tatara, Kozo, and Etsuji Okamoto. 2009. *Japan: Health System Review: Health Systems in Transition*, edited by Sara Allin, Ryozo Matsuda. Vol. 11(5): 1–164. Copenhagen: World Health Organization, European Observatory on Health Systems and Policies.

Tawaragi, Tomiko. 2008. "HBD project." Paper presented at HBD Think Tank East Meeting, July 22–23, Tokyo, Japan.

———. 2006a. "The Strategic Approach to Provide Medical Devices Speedily to Patients." Paper presented at Japan Submission Workshop, November 8–9. Tokyo, Japan.

———. 2006b. "How to Comply with Japan's Regulatory Requirements: Strategies for Success." Paper presented at Japan Submission Workshop, November 8–9. Tokyo, Japan.

Tejima, Yutaka. 1993. "Tort and Compensation in Japan: Medical Malpractice and Adverse Events from Pharmaceuticals." *University of Hawaii Law Review* 15: 728–735.

Thelen, Kathleen. 2003. "How Institutions Evolve: Insights from Comparative Historical Analysis." In *Comparative Historical Analysis in the Social Sciences*, edited by James Mahoney and Dietrich Rueschemeyer, 208–240. Cambridge: Cambridge University Press.

Today Policy Alternatives Research Institute (PARI). 2012a. "The 3rd Biomedical Innovation Workshop 2012 Report: Healthcare and Innovation—What Are the Drivers for Innovation?" Available at http://pari.u-tokyio.ac.jp/eng/event/smpl20725_infor.html (downloaded (7/18/2013).

———. 2012b. "The 2nd Biomedical Innovation Workshop 2012 Report: Toward the Realization of Biomedical Innovation in Medical Devices" (downloaded 7/18/2013).

———. 2012c. "The 5-year Strategy for Promoting Biomedical Innovation" (downloaded 6/6/2013).

Tominaga, Toshiyoshi. 2007. "MHLW's Policies on Japan's MD Clinical Trials." Paper presented at HBD West Meeting, January 11, Durham, NC.

———. 2006. "Global Harmonization Task Force Working Towards Global Harmonization in Medical Device Regulation." Conference proceedings. Paper presented at the 10th Global Harmonization Task Force (GHTF) Conference Design for Patient Safety in a Global Regulatory Model, June 29–30, Lübeck, Germany.

Tsukamoto, Hideo. 1999a. "Medical Devices-industries' Efforts to Establish Horizontal Standards of Quality." *Ikigaku* 69(9): 6–13.

———. 1999b. "The Processes Toward Global Medical Device Harmonization." *Japanese Journal of Medical Instrumentation* 69 (September 1999): 414–421. An abridged translation by Toshio Asai, January 18, 2008 (courtesy Mr. Tsukamoto, interview on January 28, 2008).

Tuohy, Caroline. 1999. *Accidental Logics: The Dynamics of Change in the Health Care Arena in the United States, Britain, and Canada*. New York: Oxford University Press.

UNDESA-ESCAP-ILO-UNEP, Expert Group Meeting on Green Growth and Green Jobs for Youth. 2012. *Comprehensive Strategy for the Rebirth of Japan—Exploring the Frontiers and Building a Country of Co-Creation*, December 12–13 session, 39–46. [United Nations Department of Economic and Social Affairs, Economic and Social Commission for Asia and the Pacific, Regional Office for Asia and the Pacific of the International Labour Organization, and United Nations Environment Program.]

United States Food and Drug Administration. "2011 FDA." Available from http://www.fda.gov.cdrh/internatinal/hdbpilot.htm.

United States International Trade Commission (USITC). 2007. *Medical Devices and Equipment: Competitive Conditions Affecting US Trade in Japan and Other Principal Foreign Markets.* Washington, DC, Publication No. 39909, Investigation Number 332–474.

United States Senate. 2001. *Testimony of Kenneth H. Keller, Chairman of the Medical Technology Leadership Forum before the Committee on Health, Education, Labor and Pensions.* Hearing on Biomedical Research: Opportunities and Innovations February 26 session, 1–6.

US and Japan MOSS Negotiating Teams. 1986a. "Report on Medical Equipment and Pharmaceuticals Market-oriented, Sector-selective (MOSS) Discussions." Washington, DC: Department of the Treasury.

———. 1986b. "MOSS Agreement on Medical Equipment and Pharmaceuticals Market-Oriented Sector-Specific Discussion by the US and the Japan MOSS Negotiating Teams." January 9: 1–76. PDF available at http://mac.doc.gov/Japan/source/menu/medpharm/ta860109.html (downloaded September 8).

Wakao, Aiko. 2007. "Japan Needs Speedier Approval for Medical Devices." *Reuters,* April 16.

Wang, Huimin. 2005. "The Case for the Patient: How Access to Leading Technology Could Improve Health Care." *ACCJ Journal* 7 (July): 1–4.

Watkins, Michael. 2004a. *The Medical Technology Industry and Japan (A).* Cambridge, MA: Harvard Business School (9-904-018).

———. 2004b. *The Medical Technology Industry and Japan (B).* Cambridge, MA: Harvard Business School (9-904-019).

Wengstrand, Megan, Takamistu Yoshida, and John C. Wocher. 2005. "Japan's Postgraduate Clinical Training: Implementation and Analysis at a Large Teaching Hospital in Japan." *Japan Hospitals* 24 (July): 3–8.

Wessel, Ramses A., and Jan Wouters. 2008. "The Phenomenon of Multilevel Regulation: Interaction between Global, EU and National Regulatory Spheres. Toward a Research Agenda." In *Multilevel Regulation and the EU: The Interplay between Global, European and National Normative Processes,* edited by Andreas Follesdal, Ramses A. Wessel and Jan Wouters, 9–47. Leiden: Martinus Nijhoff Publishers.

West, Darrell M. 2007. *Biotechnology Policy across National Boundaries: The Science-Industrial Complex.* London: Palgrave.

Wilkinson, Alan. 2007. "Gaining Reimbursement in Japan." In *Global Trends in Reimbursement of Medical Technology,* edited by Judy Rosenbloom, Jo Ellen Slurzberg, Brian Lovatt, Alan Wilkinson, Kevin Sullivan, and Duncan Fatz. Vol. CBS948, 94–123. Clinica Reports. Informa UK Ltd.

Williams, David F. 2003. "The Japanese Approach to Tissue Engineering: The Report of the Royal Academy of Engineering Mission to Japan." London: The Royal Academy of Engineering.

Wocher, John C. 2007. "Evaluating, Ranking, and Disclosing Which Hospitals, by Specialty, Are the Best in Japan—Why Not?" *Japan Hospitals* 25 (January): 3–9.

———. 2004. "Hospital Governance and the Balanced Scorecard—New Concepts for Japanese Hospitals?" *Japan Hospitals* (23) (July): 38–39.

———. 1999. "Hospital Accreditation in Japan Long Overdue?" *Japan Hospitals* 18 (July): 9–11.

Wood, Alex. 2009. "Japan All Set to Speed Up Device Approval Times." *Clinica* 1335 (March 6): 18.

World Health Organization. 2010. "WHO Western Pacific region—Japan—Country Health Information Profile." Manila, Philippines: Regional Office for the Western Pacific. Available from http://www/wpro.who.int/.

———. 2007. Sixtieth World Health Assembly. *Document WHA60.29. Agenda Item 12.19.* Geneva: WHO.

Yaginuma, Hiroshi. 2009. "Japanese MD Regulation." Paper presented at 12th Global Harmonization Conference: Realizing the Value of Technology, May 12–14, Toronto, Canada.

Yamada, Tetsuji, Chia-Ching Chen, Tadashi Yamada, I-ming Chiu, Katsunori Kondo and Chiyoe Murata. 2006. "The Japanese Healthcare Scene." Paper circulated in December 2006 through the United Kingdom-Japan-United States (UJU) health policy network established at the LSE Health in 2006.

Yamamoto, Hiroshi. 2005. "Japanese Medical Device Assessment System." Paper presented at Tapping Medical Technology to Improve Quality and Efficiency in Health Care: An International Dialogue. A Leadership Dialogue for Stakeholders and Policy Leaders from Japan and the United States, May 2–4, Washington, DC.

Yamamoto, Shuzo. 2007. "Message from the President." In *Japan Hospitals: The Journal of Japan Hospital Association* 25 (January): 1.

Yamato, Masayuki, and Teruo Okano. 2004. "Cell Sheet Engineering." *Materials Today* 7(5): 42–47.

Yang, Joseph, Masayuki Yamato, Kohji Nishida, Takeshi Ohki, Masato Kanzaki, Hidekazu Sekine, Tatsuya Shimizu, and Teruo Okano. 2006a. "Cell Delivery in Regenerative Medicine: the Cell Sheet Engineering Approach." *Journal of Controlled Release: Science Direct* 116(206): 193–203.

———. 2006b. "Corneal Epithelial Stem Cell Delivery Using Cell Sheet Engineering: Not Lost in Transplantation." *Journal of Drug Targeting* 14(7): 471–482.

Yeo, Ashley. 2013. "Japan's Device Drug Regulator Urges Focus on English Language for a Global Industry." August 8. http://www.rajpharma.com/productsector/medicaldevices/Japans-devucedrug-regulator (received August 8, 2013).

———. 2010. "The Regulator's Chance to Catch Up with Science." *RAJ Devices*, http://www.rajdevices.com (accessed September 30, 2010).

Index